Otolaryngologic Trauma

Editor

SYDNEY C. BUTTS

OTOLARYNGOLOGIC CLINICS OF NORTH AMERICA

www.oto.theclinics.com

Consulting Editor
SUJANA S. CHANDRASEKHAR

December 2023 • Volume 56 • Number 6

ELSEVIER

1600 John F. Kennedy Boulevard • Suite 1800 • Philadelphia, Pennsylvania, 19103-2899

http://www.oto.theclinics.com

OTOLARYNGOLOGIC CLINICS OF NORTH AMERICA Volume 56, Number 6
December 2023 ISSN 0030-6665, ISBN-13: 978-0-443-18371-3

Editor: Stacy Eastman
Developmental Editor: Malvika Shah

Otolaryngologic Clinics of North America (ISSN 0030-6665) is published bimonthly by Elsevier, Inc., 360 Park Avenue South, New York, NY 10010-1710. Months of issue are February, April, June, August, October, and December. Business and Editorial Offices: 1600 John F. Kennedy Blvd., Suite 1800, Philadelphia, PA 19103-2899. Customer Service Office: 6277 Sea Harbor Drive, Orlando, FL 32887-4800. Periodicals postage paid at New York, NY and additional mailing offices. Subscription prices are $468.00 per year (US individuals), $1117.00 per year (US institutions), $100.00 per year (US & Canadian student/resident), $599.00 per year (Canadian individuals), $1416.00 per year (Canadian institutions), $653.00 per year (international individuals), $1416.00 per year (international institutions), $270.00 per year (international student/resident). Foreign air speed delivery is included in all *Clinics'* subscription prices. All prices are subject to change without notice. **POSTMASTER:** Send address changes to *Otolaryngologic Clinics of North America*, Elsevier Health Sciences Division, Subscription Customer Service, 3251 Riverport Lane, Maryland Heights, MO 63043. **Telephone: 1-800-654-2452 (U.S. and Canada); 314-447-8871 (outside U.S. and Canada). Fax: 314-447-8029. E-mail: journalscustomerservice-usa@elsevier.com (for print support); journalsonlinesupport-usa@elsevier.com (for online support).**

Reprints. For copies of 100 or more of articles in this publication, please contact the Commercial Reprints Department, Elsevier Inc., 360 Park Avenue South, New York, NY 10010-1710. Tel.: 212-633-3874; Fax: 212-633-3820; E-mail: reprints@elsevier.com.

Otolaryngologic Clinics of North America is also published in Spanish by McGraw-Hill Interamericana Editores S.A., P.O. Box 5-237, 06500 Mexico D.F., Mexico.

Otolaryngologic Clinics of North America is covered in *MEDLINE/PubMed (Index Medicus), Current Contents/Clinical Medicine, Excerpta Medica, BIOSIS, Science Citation Index,* and *ISI/BIOMED.*

Contributors

CONSULTING EDITOR

SUJANA S. CHANDRASEKHAR, MD, FAAO-HNS, FAOS, FACS
Consulting Editor, *Otolaryngologic Clinics of North America*, President, American
Otological Society, Past President, American Academy of Otolaryngology–Head and Neck
Surgery, Partner, ENT & Allergy Associates, LLP, Clinical Professor, Department of
Otolaryngology–Head and Neck Surgery, Zucker School of Medicine at Hofstra/Northwell,
Clinical Associate Professor, Department of Otolaryngology–Head and Neck Surgery,
Icahn School of Medicine at Mount Sinai, New York, New York

EDITOR

SYDNEY C. BUTTS, MD, FACS
Interim Chair, Associate Professor, Chief, Facial Plastic and Reconstructive Surgery,
Department of Otolaryngology, SUNY Downstate Health Sciences University, Department
of Otolaryngology, Kings County Hospital Center, Brooklyn, New York

AUTHORS

SELENA E. BRIGGS, MD, PhD, MBA, FACS
Associate Professor, Department of Otolaryngology–Head and Neck Surgery, MedStar
Georgetown University Hospital, Vice Chair, Department of Otolaryngology–Head and
Neck Surgery, MedStar Washington Hospital Center, Washington, DC

SARA ABU-GHANEM, MD, MmedSc
Assistant Professor, Laryngology and Bronchoesophagology, Department of
Otolaryngology, SUNY Downstate, Maimonides Health, Brooklyn, New York

DANE M. BARRETT, MD, MBA
Assistant Professor, Department of Head and Neck Surgery, Communication Sciences,
Duke South Yellow Zone, Durham, North Carolina

ANTHONY BOTROS, MD
Department of Otolaryngology–Head and Neck Surgery, Emory University School of
Medicine, Atlanta, Georgia

JENNINGS RUSSELL BOYETTE, MD
Department of Otolaryngology–Head and Neck Surgery, University of Arkansas for
Medical Sciences, Little Rock, Arkansas

SHARON BRANGMAN, MD
Department of Geriatrics, SUNY Upstate University Hospital, Syracuse, New York

SARA BRESSLER MD
Louisiana State University Health Sciences Center-New Orleans, New Orleans, Louisiana

SYDNEY C. BUTTS, MD, FACS
Interim Chair, Associate Professor, Chief, Facial Plastic and Reconstructive Surgery, Department of Otolaryngology, SUNY Downstate Health Sciences University, Department of Otolaryngology, Kings County Hospital Center, Brooklyn, New York

TYLER G. CHAN, BS
Emory University School of Medicine, Atlanta, Georgia

TZU-HSUAN CHENG, MD
Resident, Department of Anesthesiology, State University of New York Downstate Health Sciences University, Brooklyn, New York

NATALYA CHERNICHENKO, MD
Associate Professor, Department of Otolaryngology, SUNY Downstate Health Sciences University, Department of Otolaryngology, Kings County Hospital Center, Brooklyn, New York

NICHOLAS W. CLARK, MD
Department of Head and Neck Surgery, Communication Sciences, Duke South Yellow Zone, Durham, North Carolina

JAMES COCHRAN, MD
Resident, Department of Otolaryngology, SUNY Downstate Health Sciences University, Brooklyn, New York

WENYU DENG, MD
Department of Ophthalmology, SUNY Downstate Medical Center, Department of Ophthalmology, Kings County Medical Center, Brooklyn, New York

ANTOINETTE ESCE, MD
Division of Otolaryngology–Head and Neck Surgery, Department of Surgery, PGY-4, Department of Surgery ENT 1, University of New Mexico, Albuquerque, New Mexico

ANNA CELESTE GIBSON, MD
Department of Otolaryngology–Head and Neck Surgery, University of Arkansas for Medical Sciences, Little Rock, Arkansas

JENNIFER GOTTFRIED, BS
Medical Student, SUNY Downstate Health Sciences University, College of Medicine, Brooklyn, New York

JAMES M. HAMILTON, MD
Department of Otolaryngology–Head and Neck Surgery, Emory University School of Medicine, Department of Otolaryngology–Head and Neck Surgery, Grady Memorial Hospital, Atlanta, Georgia

DANIEL HAWKINS, DMD
Department of Oral and Maxillofacial Surgery, Virginia Commonwealth University, Richmond, Virginia

OSWALDO A. HENRIQUEZ, MD
Department of Otolaryngology–Head and Neck Surgery, Emory University School of Medicine, Atlanta, Georgia

NICKISA M. HODGSON, MD
Assistant Professor, Department of Ophthalmology, SUNY Downstate Medical Center, Department of Ophthalmology, Kings County Medical Center, Brooklyn, New York

JAMES DIXON JOHNS, MD
Department of Otolaryngology–Head and Neck Surgery, MedStar Georgetown University Hospital, Department of Otolaryngology–Head and Neck Surgery, MedStar Washington Hospital Center, Washington, DC

RUSSEL R. KAHMKE, MD, MMCi
Assistant Professor, Department of Head and Neck Surgery, Communication Sciences, Duke South Yellow Zone, Durham, North Carolina

ALEXANDREA KIM, MD
Department of Otolaryngology–Head and Neck Surgery, Emory University School of Medicine, Atlanta, Georgia

PETER KWAK, MD
Department of Otolaryngology–Head and Neck Surgery, Virginia Commonwealth University, Richmond, Virginia

CLARA LEE, MD
PYG4, Department of Otolaryngology–Head and Neck Surgery, Columbia University Irving Medical Center, New York, New York

THOMAS S. LEE, MD
Department of Otolaryngology–Head and Neck Surgery, Virginia Commonwealth University, Associate Professor, Division Chief of Facial Reconstruction and Trauma Surgery, Facial Plastic and Reconstructive Microsurgery, Head and Neck Cancer Surgery, Skull Base Surgery, Department of Otolaryngology–Head and Neck Surgery, Virginia Commonwealth University Hospital, Richmond, Virginia

DANIEL J. MEARA, MS, MD, DMD, MHCDS, FACS
Attending Surgeon, Department of Oral and Maxillofacial Surgery and Hospital Dentistry, Chair, Christiana Care Health System, Wilmington, Delaware; Affiliate Faculty, Department of Physical Therapy, University of Delaware, Newark, Delaware

DUNCAN A. MEIKLEJOHN, MD
Division of Otolaryngology–Head and Neck Surgery, Department of Surgery, PGY-2, Department of Surgery ENT 1, University of New Mexico, Albuquerque, New Mexico

MATTHEW MENDELSOHN, MD
Resident, Department of Otolaryngology, State University of New York Downstate Health Sciences University, Brooklyn, New York

TYLER BRANCH MERRILL, MD
Department of Otolaryngology–Head and Neck Surgery, University of Arkansas for Medical Sciences, Little Rock, Arkansas

CHARLES E. MOORE, MD
Department of Otolaryngology–Head and Neck Surgery, Emory University School of Medicine, Department of Otolaryngology–Head and Neck Surgery, Grady Memorial Hospital, Atlanta, Georgia

LISA MORRIS MD
Assistant Professor, Louisiana State University Health Sciences Center-New Orleans, New Orleans, Louisiana

CLAUDE NGANZEU, MD
Division of Otolaryngology–Head and Neck Surgery, Department of Surgery, PGY-2, Department of Surgery ENT 1, University of New Mexico, Albuquerque, New Mexico

MICHAEL NUARA, MD
Division of Facial Plastic and Reconstructive Surgery, Virginia Mason Franciscan Health, Seattle, Washington

RADHA P. PANDYA, BS
Department of Ophthalmology, SUNY Downstate Medical Center, Brooklyn, New York

KOUROSH PARHAM, MD
Department of Otolaryngology–Head and Neck Surgery, University of Connecticut, Farmington, Connecticut

RADHIKA PATEL, MD
Student, State University of New York Downstate Health Sciences University, Brooklyn, New York

SACHIN S. PAWAR, MD
Division Chief and Fellowship Director, Facial Plastic and Reconstructive Surgery, Department of Otolaryngology and Communication Sciences, Surgical Medical Informatics Officer, Froedtert & the Medical College of Wisconsin, Associate Professor, Medical College of Wisconsin, Milwaukee, Wisconsin

CORINNE PITTMAN, MD
Department of Otolaryngology–Head and Neck Surgery, MedStar Georgetown University Hospital, Department of Otolaryngology–Head and Neck Surgery, MedStar Washington Hospital Center, Washington, DC

DAVID B. POWERS, MD, DMD
Professor, Division of Plastic, Maxillofacial, and Oral Surgery, Department of Surgery, Durham, North Carolina

JACEY PUDNEY, MD
Department of Geriatrics, SUNY Upstate University Hospital, Syracuse, New York

THEODORE SCHUMAN, MD
Department of Otolaryngology–Head and Neck Surgery, Virginia Commonwealth University, Richmond, Virginia

LUCY L. SHI, MD
Division of Facial Plastic and Reconstructive Surgery, Virginia Mason Franciscan Health, Seattle, Washington

H. STEVEN SIMS, MD, FACS
Francis L. Lederer Professor of Otolaryngology–Head and Neck Surgery, University of Illinois Hospital and Health Service Systems, Chicago, Illinois

DIMITRIOS SISMANIS, MD
Virginia Oculofacial Surgeons, Oculoplastic Surgery, Richmond, Virginia

ABIGAIL B. THOMAS, MD
Department of Otolaryngology and Communication Sciences, Medical College of Wisconsin, Milwaukee, Wisconsin

OSCAR TRUJILLO, MD, MS
Director of Cosmetic Facial Plastic Surgery, Assistant Professor, Department of Otolaryngology–Head and Neck Surgery, Columbia University Irving Medical Center, New York, New York

NIMA VAHIDI, MD
Department of Otolaryngology–Head and Neck Surgery, Virginia Commonwealth University, Richmond, Virginia

ROHAN R. WALVEKAR, MD
Clinical Professor, Mervin L. Trail Endowed Chair in Head and Neck Oncology, Director-Salivary Endoscopy Service, Department of Otolaryngology–Head and Neck Surgery, Louisiana State University Health Sciences Center, New Orleans, Louisiana

CHARLES R. WOODARD, MD
Associate Professor, Department of Head and Neck Surgery, Communication Sciences, Duke South Yellow Zone, Durham, North Carolina

SAMRAT WORAH, MD
Assistant Professor, Department of Anesthesiology, State University of New York Downstate Health Sciences University, Brooklyn, New York

Contents

The facial trauma surgeon will see a variety of facial injuries. Recognition of emergency cases and proper intervention is and this article aims to highlight those cases and the respective proper interventions.

Penetrating injury to the head and neck accounts for a minority of trauma but significant morbidity in the US civilian population. The 3-zone anatomical framework has historically guided evaluation and management; however, the most current evidence-based protocols favor a no-zone, systems-based approach. In stable patients, a thorough physical examination and noninvasive imaging should be prioritized, with surgical exploration of the head and neck reserved for certain circumstances. Diagnostic and management decisions should be tailored to the mechanism of injury, history, physical examination, experience of personnel, availability of equipment, and clinical judgment.

 Video content accompanies this article at http://www.oto.theclinics.com.

This review will focus on the key steps in the recognition of parotid gland and duct injuries focusing on the important steps needed at the initial assessment. Management planning is presented in the way that trauma surgeons interact with patients, highlighting the important parts of the informed consent conversation followed by the key information that must be communicated to the anesthesia and operating room teams, which ensures proper monitoring and equipment needs are in place. Short-term and long-term outcomes for patients with persistent sequelae of the trauma and their management are reviewed.

article is a comprehensive review of standard and minimally invasive approaches, with description of techniques and pros and cons for their use.

Nasal fractures are very common. The literature describes early intervention (<14 days) with closed techniques as cost-effective, minimizing the need for possible secondary surgeries and improved early patient satisfaction. However, the authors observe a measurably high rate of subsequent open treatment after closed treatment, particularly where there is significant septal involvement in the fracture. Moreover, delayed intervention (>3 months) with an open approach has many advantages over early closed technique, including lower revision rate, improved ability for rigid fixation and support, and the ability to correct severe dorsal or caudal L-strut deformities, nasal valve issues, and severe nasal bony deviation/deformities.

Orbital floor fractures are a common manifestation of facial trauma that is encountered by ophthalmology, otolaryngology, and oral maxillofacial specialists. Surgical intervention is required emergently in cases of tissue entrapment and less urgently in cases of presenting with persistent diplopia, enophthalmos greater than 2 mm, and/or fractures involving greater than 50% of the orbital floor. Surgical management is a debated topic with differing opinions among surgeons regarding timing of repair, type of implant, and surgical approach.

The goal of mandibular fracture management is to restore form and function. Maxillomandibular fixation, elastic occlusal guidance, and postoperative physiotherapy are essential elements to optimizing outcomes. Restoration of premorbid occlusion is paramount. Thus, an expert understanding of occlusion, coupled with the application of maxillomandibular techniques to achieve bony reduction with idealized dental occlusion, is required in the proper management of mandible fractures. Postoperatively, complete recovery initially requires elastic occlusal guidance followed by jaw range of motion physiotherapy. Bone healing, an idealized occlusion, and normal jaw range of motion signal success via the restoration of form and function.

This article provides a review of the current technologies available in the preoperative and intraoperative management of complex and secondary maxillofacial trauma reconstruction. These patients present a unique challenge for which the advancement of imaging technologies, patient-specific modeling and implants, and intraoperative imaging and navigation can play an important role to improve their post-treatment outcomes.

Mandible fracture management has evolved dramatically. Therefore, the variety of surgical complications associated with mandibular fractures, and their incidences, have continued to change as well. This article aims to assess the most common and most concerning complications that can occur secondary to management of mandibular fractures by examining categories of complication types. This article also explores factors and techniques associated with reduced rates of complications as well as the management of complications.

Craniomaxillofacial trauma is a challenging entity to manage effectively and often necessitates serial evaluation and treatment. A multidisciplinary team is best served to evaluate and treat these complex injury patterns with the use of necessary adjuncts, such as neuronavigation, intraoperative imaging, custom implant use, and virtual surgical planning. Complications of facial trauma can present at a spectrum of time points and manifest in a variety of manners and as such patients should be observed closely and longitudinally. Although not all complications and secondary deformities can be avoided, this article highlights some common pitfalls and our unique management strategies.

The pediatric patient population has unique anatomic characteristics that bring challenges and increased risk to management. The purpose of this article is to guide the head and neck trauma surgeon in decision making for the treatment of pediatric head and neck trauma with an emphasis on facial fracture management.

Craniofacial trauma in the geriatric population is increasing as our population ages. Due to loss of bone quality and medical comorbidities, injuries for minor trauma can be severe. A more extensive medical evaluation is usually warranted in this population before proceeding with surgery. In addition, unique surgical considerations exist in the repair of atrophic and edentulous bony fractures. Some quality improvement measures have already been undertaken but more is needed to help standardize care in this vulnerable population.

OTOLARYNGOLOGIC CLINICS OF NORTH AMERICA

SERIES OF RELATED INTEREST

Facial Plastic Surgery Clinics
Available at: https://www.facialplastic.theclinics.com/

Foreword

Caring for the Patient with Otolaryngologic Trauma Is a Complex Matter

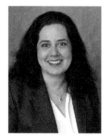

Sujana S. Chandrasekhar, MD, FAAO-HNS, FAOS, FACS
Consulting Editor

Craniomaxillofacial trauma occurs in isolation or in combination with other serious injuries, including intracranial, spinal, and upper- and lower-body injuries.[1] Facial fractures can be disabling injuries that may be a major cause of expensive treatment and rehabilitation requirements, temporary or lifelong morbidity, and loss of human productivity. Despite the utilization of sophisticated diagnostics and surgical treatment approaches, particularly in high-resource health care systems, occult facial fractures, often seen with low-energy mechanisms, are frequent and are often missed. This can cause delay in management and potentially result in suboptimal outcomes.

In an Austrian study of 14,654 patients with 35,129 injuries treated at a single Department of Cranio-Maxillofacial and Oral Surgery over a 15-year period, the following was seen.[1] Older people were more prone to soft tissue lesions with a rising risk of 2.1% per year older, equal in men and women. Younger patients were at higher risk of dentoalveolar trauma with an increase of 4.4% per year younger, and this was 19.6% higher for women. The risk of sustaining facial bone fractures increased each year by 4.6% and was 66.4% times higher in men. A total of 2550 patients (17.4%) suffered 3834 concomitant injuries of other body parts.

It is interesting and informative to look at this problem from a Global Burden of Disease standpoint.[2] In 2017, there were an estimated 7,538,663 new facial fractures globally. Between 1990 and 2017, the global age-standardized incidence rate did not change significantly, and it was on average 98 per 100,000 in 2017. The global age-standardized prevalence of facial fractures was 23 per 100,000 in 2017, or approximately 1,819,732 ($\pm$200,000) individuals globally living with any disability from a facial fracture. From 1990 to 2017, there was a significant decrease in the age-standardized prevalence of facial fractures by an average of 2.8%.

Otolaryngol Clin N Am 56 (2023) xv–xvii
https://doi.org/10.1016/j.otc.2023.08.005
0030-6665/23/© 2023 Published by Elsevier Inc.

oto.theclinics.com

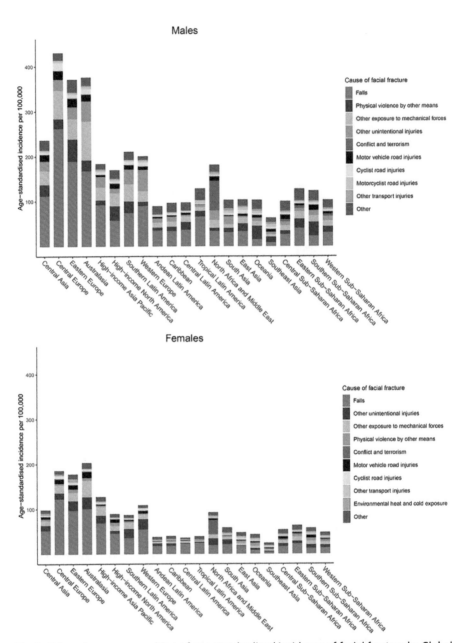

Fig. 1. External cause composition of age-standardized incidence of facial fracture by Global Burden of Disease region. (*From* Lalloo R, Lucchesi LR, Bisignano C, et al, Epidemiology of facial fractures: incidence, prevalence and years lived with disability estimates from the Global Burden of Disease 2017 study. Injury Prevention 2020;26: i27-i35, figure 5.)

Globally, facial fractures result from myriad causes, as seen in **Fig. 1**. Falls, motor vehicle injuries, other mechanical forces, and physical violence are the most common across the globe, with terrorism prevalent in North Africa and the Middle East. The United States has a unique experience with firearms injuries. Between 2009 and

2017, there were approximately 120,232 people injured by firearms per year, or 329 every day.[3] For every person who died from a firearm injury, there were another two people who survived. Even "rubber bullets" used in crowd control can cause life-altering trauma. Dr Lilun Li, then an otolaryngology resident, detailed this in an op-ed article she wrote and on my video show, "She's On Call."[4,5]

We tend to associate disability-associated life-years or years lived with disability (YLDs) with chronic illness, but this statistic is meaningful when considering facial trauma. Globally, facial fractures caused 117,402 YLDs in 2017, with an average disability weight of 6.5%. This means that on average each person with a prevalent facial fracture lost 6.5% of their normal health status. The number is significantly lower in high- and high-middle-income countries and significantly higher in middle- and low-income countries.

Management of the patient with otolaryngologic trauma involves compassionate, comprehensive, often team-based care, including otolaryngic, facial plastic, orbital, dental, neurologic, and airway management. I commend Dr Sydney Butts on assembling this likewise comprehensive issue of *Otolaryngologic Clinics of North America* on this subject. Her call to action in terms of public health measures to protect our communities, and her reference to the "sense of duty" that we feel when caring for our patients should give us all hope for the future.

Sujana S. Chandrasekhar, MD, FAAO-HNS, FAOS, FACS
Consulting Editor, Otolaryngologic Clinics of North America
President, American Otological Society
Past President, American Academy of Otolaryngology-Head and Neck Surgery
Partner, ENT & Allergy Associates, LLP
Clinical Professor, Department of Otolaryngology-Head and Neck Surgery, Zucker
School of Medicine at Hofstra-Northwell
Clinical Associate Professor, Department of Otolaryngology-Head and Neck Surgery,
Icahn School of Medicine at Mount Sinai
18 East 48th Street, 2nd Floor
New York, NY 10017, USA

E-mail address:
ssc@nyotology.com

REFERENCES

1. Kraft A, Abermann E, Stigler R, et al. Craniomaxillofacial trauma: synopsis of 14,654 cases with 35,129 injuries in 15 years. Craniomaxillofac Trauma Reconstr 2012;5(1):41–50.
2. Lalloo R, Lucchesi LR, Bisignano C, et al. Epidemiology of facial fractures: incidence, prevalence and years lived with disability estimates from the Global Burden of Disease 2017 study. Inj Prev 2020;26:i27–35.
3. Kaufman EJ, Wiebe DJ, Xiong RA, et al. Epidemiologic trends in fatal and nonfatal firearm injuries in the US, 2009-2017. JAMA Intern Med 2021;181(2):237–44.
4. Li L. Opinion Rubber bullets are touted as a 'safe alternative.' My patient's wound tells a different story. Washington Post, June 4, 2020. Available at: https://www.washingtonpost.com/opinions/2020/06/04/rubber-bullets-are-touted-safe-alternative-my-patients-wound-tells-different-story/. Accessed August 6, 2023.
5. She's On Call episode 2, aired Sunday, June 21, 2020. Available at: https://www.youtube.com/watch?v=alelQZtnGFM. Accessed August 6, 2023.

Preface

Management of Otolaryngic Trauma: Assessing Current Risks, Care Needs, and Evidence-Based Treatment

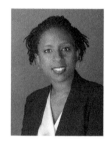

Sydney C. Butts, MD, FACS
Editor

Management of trauma patients has always been an important part of the otolaryngologist's surgical and teaching mission. More recently, this mission has a significance that has grown. Past public health initiatives, including seat belt laws, automobiles equipped with airbags, and greater helmet use by bicyclists, have successfully decreased the rates and severity of many types of head and neck trauma. Current day risks now expose the public to trauma that should drive public health responses similar to those implemented decades ago that successfully addressed motor vehicle and transportation injuries. Risks from interpersonal violence from gun use and other weapons are front of mind for all surgeons who manage head and neck trauma.[1] Population changes in the United States must also be considered in the context of trauma risk. The demographics of facial trauma have traditionally shown the highest rates among younger men. The aging population in the United States compels a focus on the increasing percentage of Americans over 65 years of age who are also victims of head and neck trauma, often from falls. Cities addressing automobile traffic with "green" efforts that encourage increased use of bicycles and scooters also need to address the vulnerability of these riders to trauma.[2]

The management of head and neck trauma can be demanding but ultimately an extremely rewarding experience. McCusker and Schmalbach[3] reported results of a survey distributed to recent otolaryngology residency graduates to ascertain the percentage who manage trauma patients and the motivating factors to do so. Eight-five percent of respondents indicated that they treat patients with maxillofacial trauma, and 64% identified trauma management as a desirable part of their practice, with

Otolaryngol Clin N Am 56 (2023) xix–xx
https://doi.org/10.1016/j.otc.2023.07.006
0030-6665/23/© 2023 Published by Elsevier Inc.

"sense of duty" being a leading reason. Respondents assessed themselves as well trained in most areas of facial trauma. The dedication of otolaryngologists early in their careers to trauma management is important and speaks to the strong training and mentorship that residency training programs are offering.

In this issue of *Otolaryngology Clinics of North America*, there is an emphasis on the management of complex trauma cases, especially addressing complications or secondary deformity and how technology can be an aid. Advancements in treatment approaches and identification of treatment debates that compare outcomes are discussed in several articles. For instance, the debate between outpatient or inpatient orbital fracture management; the utility of virtual surgical planning, intraoperative CT, and types of maxillo-mandibular fixation are analyzed in terms of patient outcomes, cost, and impact on operative time.

Head and neck trauma has traditionally included management with other surgical specialties—plastic surgery, oral maxillofacial surgery, and ophthalmology—resulting in opportunities for multidisciplinary care management. The background of the authors in this issue reflects the multispecialty nature of head and neck trauma management. This was done intentionally to emphasize the complexity of care management and the importance of communication among specialists to achieve the best outcomes. In addition, holistic patient approaches are emphasized with attention to the perioperative assessments that may impact trauma treatment outcomes.

Sydney C. Butts, MD, FACS
Department of Otolaryngology
SUNY Downstate Health Sciences Center
450 Clarkson Avenue, Box 126
Brooklyn, NY 11203, USA

E-mail address:
sydney.butts@downstate.edu

REFERENCES

1. Bauchner H, Rivara FP, Bonow RO, et al. Death by gun violence—a public health crisis. JAMA Psychiatry 2017;74(12):1195–6.
2. Lee KH, Chou HJ. Facial fractures in road cyclists. Aust Dent J 2008;53(3):246–9.
3. McCusker SB, Schmalbach CE. The otolaryngologist's cost in treating facial trauma: American Academy of Otolaryngology–Head and Neck Surgery survey. Otolaryngol Head Neck Surg 2012;146(3):366–71.

Soft Tissue Trauma
Critical Recognition and Timing of Intervention in Emergency Presentations

Nicholas W. Clark, MD[a], Dane M. Barrett, MD, MBA[a],
Russel R. Kahmke, MD, MMCi[a], David B. Powers, MD, DMD[b],
Charles R. Woodard, MD[a],*

KEYWORDS

• Facial trauma • Laceration • Avulsion • Soft tissue

KEY POINTS

• Repair of auricular avulsion should consider the need for secondary repair and not hinder secondary repair.
• Complete facial nerve transection should be repaired primarily and eye care is critical in the prevention of secondary injury in any degree of facial nerve injury.
• Nasal, auricular, and eyelid injuries should be repaired in layers and attention paid to meticulous closure to prevent cosmetic deformity.

INTRODUCTION

All trauma patients should be evaluated using the systematic trauma protocols as established by the Advanced Trauma Life Support (ATLS) program. The primary survey of a trauma patient focuses on evaluating the Airway, Breathing, and Circulation (ABC).[1] All wounds should be thoroughly irrigated, and appropriate tetanus prophylaxis should be given. In cases of frank contamination, irrigation with dilute soap solution may be considered. Antiseptic solutions can risk cellular injury of traumatized tissue.[2] The use of antibiotics in facial soft tissue injuries depends on the specific injury severity, mechanism, wound contamination, and surgeon preference.[3] Studies have shown no benefit for prophylactic antibiotics in cases of superficial skin lacerations.[4] However, they may provide benefits in cases of immunocompromised patients, grossly contaminated wounds, delayed wound closure, patients with a high risk of endocarditis, and high-velocity gunshot wounds.[4] Many facial soft tissue injuries

[a] Department of Head and Neck Surgery, Communication Sciences, Duke South Yellow Zone, 4000 DUMC Box 3805, Durham, NC 27710, USA; [b] Division of Plastic, Maxillofacial, and Oral Surgery, Department of Surgery, DUMC 2955, Durham, NC 27710, USA
* Corresponding author.
E-mail address: Charles.woodard@duke.edu

Otolaryngol Clin N Am 56 (2023) 1003–1012
https://doi.org/10.1016/j.otc.2023.05.009
0030-6665/23/Published by Elsevier Inc.
oto.theclinics.com

can be repaired under local anesthesia, and specific regional blocks will be discussed later in discussion. Skeletal trauma will not be the focus of this article but should be included in the facial trauma evaluation.

DISCUSSION
Complete or Partial Auricular Avulsion

The ear, with its intricate vasculature and thin, delicate skin, can make avulsion repair, regardless of the preceding mechanism, challenging; their position on the head makes any deformity more visible to others. Auricular injury commonly occurs from motor vehicle trauma and auricular injury typically involves more than 2/3 of the total ear.[5–8]

The first step in evaluating auricular trauma is wound debridement (including pressured irrigation) and cleansing avulsed segments with 10% povidone-iodine.[7] A completely avulsed segment should be wrapped in gauze, placed in a plastic bag, and stored on ice (4°C).[7] Prior studies have shown that an auricle stored in this fashion can last for many hours, with one study showing successful reimplantation after 33 hours.[9] The auricle is supplied by branches of the superficial temporal artery and post-auricular artery, which communicate via a helical arcade. Due to vascular redundancy, the auricle can survive if one single vessel from either artery is intact.[10] The auricular cartilage derives its blood supply from the perichondrium supplied by thin skin covering.[11]

The choice of repair technique should consider the possible need for secondary reconstruction, which can be negatively influenced by an injury to the surrounding periauricular skin during the initial repair technique. Care should be taken to address auricular hematoma via drainage and prevent occurrence after repair. The authors prefer full-thickness absorbable quilting suture. An ear wick should be placed if injuries extend into the external auditory canal to prevent canal stenosis. An example of a significant auricular injury is shown in **Fig. 1**, where primary repair, **Fig. 2**, was performed and trimmed non-absorbable nasal packing was placed in the canal to prevent canal stenosis.

A systematic review by Gailey and colleagues found microvascular repair and those auricular injuries in which partial avulsion occurred tended to provide better

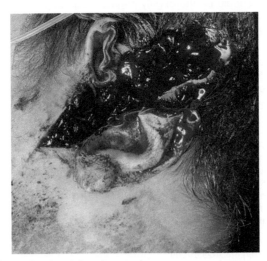

Fig. 1. Auricular laceration involving the canal.

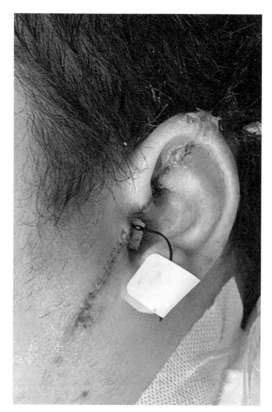

Fig. 2. Auricular laceration repair with canal stent.

outcomes.[5] Microvascular repair was shown to have superior results in additional studies but demanded intensive perioperative and post-operative treatment (including multi-day hospital stay, leech therapy, and need for blood transfusions).[8,11] Gailey and colleagues evaluated seven different reattachment techniques (microvascular repair, simple reattachment, local flap, pocket technique, temporoparietal fascia (TPF) flap, platysma myocutaneous flap, Baudet method) and concluded that microvascular repair and simple reattachment were the better options by the aesthetic outcome and mentioned these techniques did not disrupt post-auricular skin and therefore did not preclude later reconstruction if needed.[5] Antibiotics are commonly prescribed in the postoperative period[8] but adequate evidence supporting their use is lacking.[11]

The temporoparietal fascia flap (TPF flap) is regarded as a viable reconstructive option that can be employed when other local vascular options are not available. Reconstruction with a TPF flap can be difficult. TPF flap should be employed in a delayed fashion, and only for those surgeons with extensive auricular reconstruction experience.[5,6] Non-microvascular techniques such as the TPF flap and pocket tend to result in distortion and shrinkage of the auricle due to fibrosis and cartilage resorption. This can make secondary reconstruction with rib graft or implant more difficult.[8,11] In cases of total auricular avulsion, microvascular repair is recommended if certain conditions are met. First, the amputated auricle must be available for reimplantation and suitable vessels must be identified on examination. Second, the facility must have microvascular capabilities. Finally, the patient must consent to an extended hospital stay and to blood transfusions.[11] In cases of partial avulsion, primary repair is recommended as even small millimeter pedicles are successful.[2] For those cases where soft tissue reconstruction cannot be achieved collaboration with an anaplastologist for prosthesis is a viable option.[12]

Facial Nerve Injury

The facial nerve provides innervation to all muscles of facial expression. After exiting the stylomastoid foramen, the facial nerve enters the parotid gland and bifurcates into temporofacial and cervicofacial branches at the pes anserinus.[13] The nerve continues to further divide into the temporal, zygomatic, buccal, mandibular, and cervical branches distally. After the nerve enters the parotid gland, its course becomes increasingly superficial.[13]

Injury to the facial nerve from soft tissue trauma can occur from penetrating or blunt trauma. The location of the injury dictates the presentation. A physical exam should be performed, assessing all branches of the facial nerve as soon as possible after the injury to obtain a baseline. Delayed paralysis or post-injury edema can make the assessment of facial motion more difficult. Injuries anterior to a vertical line drawn inferiorly from the lateral canthus are often not explored, as branches of the nerve at this point can be challenging to find and repair due to their small diameter.[14] Various facial nerve grading systems exist. Regardless of which grading system is used, clear and detailed documentation of the involved branches and degree of the deficit is most important.

Various nerve function tests exist. Most are designed to test the facial nerve at the main trunk as it exits the stylomastoid foramen. Electromyography (EMG) is considered most useful for distal or transection injuries because the test evaluates electrical activity produced by skeletal muscle.[14] Normal muscle function will demonstrate intact motor unit action potentials. Acute denervation injuries will demonstrate spontaneous fibrillation potentials. During reinnervation, polyphasic action potentials are seen.[14] The ideal timing for EMG is after Wallerian degeneration of the nerve has occurred (typically 72 hours after injury[14]) and ideally at around 14 days.[14] Electroneuronography (ENOG) is another test that can be helpful, ENOG records action potentials at the distal facial muscles. It is most useful when used in the first six days after paralysis and when performed serially. Serial testing makes ENOG less practical than EMG.[15]

When the facial nerve is completely transected, direct repair will provide the best chance of recovery and outcome. Multiple options are available in cases where direct repair is not possible. Techniques for dynamic facial reanimation can be broadly grouped into neural or muscular procedures.[14] Neural approaches consist of direct repair, cable grafting, and nerve transposition. Muscular approaches include tendon or muscle transpositions such as the temporalis tendon transfer. In chronically denervated patients, free tissue transfer with both muscle and nerve may be required to restore dynamic facial movement.

Most important in the acute phase of facial nerve injury is the prevention of additional complications. For this reason, eye care is critical. Eye care consists of saline eye drops every 1-2 hours as needed, eye ointment nightly, moisture chamber or eyelid taped closed at bedtime to prevent corneal desiccation and subsequent complications, including blindness.

Large Scalp Lacerations/Soft Tissue Avulsion

Soft tissue avulsions encompass cases of trauma where tissue loss ranges from minimal to complete. The anatomic region of the avulsion will dictate optimal repair. If partially avulsed, examination for capillary refill and bleeding from wound edges can help determine viability. Tissue should be debrided conservatively, even if non-viable; at the very least it can serve as a biological dressing.

Scalp examination is critical in the facial trauma patient as hair can mask the severity of the injury. This can be further masked by supine positioning and cervical spine immobilization. Therefore, examining the entire scalp comprehensively, including under the cervical collar (while stabilizing the cervical spine) is essential. Thorough irrigation is vital in accurately assessing the extent of scalp lacerations. The authors recommend mild soap and high-volume saline irrigation, similar to washing one's hair when bathing. Hemostasis is critical in scalp laceration management, as well as the placement of drains in cases of large scalp lacerations to prevent hematoma. Electrocautery should be minimized and performed judiciously to avoid causing alopecia.[2] Generally, hair shaving is not recommended prior to scalp laceration repair and may increase the risk of infection.[16] The scalp should be closed in layers (periosteum, galea, dermis) with the goal of tension-free closure. Surgical staples are recommended for the closure of the superficial layer. In cases where tension-free closure is difficult, scoring of the galeal layer can facilitate the closure of high-tension areas.[2] In cases of large scalp lacerations with tissue loss, primary closure can sometimes be achieved. In these specific cases, perforating towel clamps can help approximate the tissue temporarily while the deep layers are being closed. The authors have found the use of a towel clamp valuable in cases of tissue loss, and clamps are typically applied for 10 to 20 minutes. In cases of total scalp avulsion, microvascular repair by an experienced microvascular surgeon is recommended,[17] giving the best chance of success and cosmetic outcome. **Fig. 3** depicts a large scalp injury that was repaired in layers and a drain was placed.

Nasal Lacerations: Full-Thickness or Cartilage Exposure

Nasal lacerations should be copiously irrigated and closed meticulously. Local anesthetic should be applied to achieve nasal block. The nose is innervated by the first and second division of the trigeminal nerve, which supplies innervation to the lateral nasal sidewall (infratrochlear nerve), the nasal dorsum and nasal tip (external branch of the anterior ethmoidal nerve), and the lower third of the nose (second division of the trigeminal nerve).[18] A nasal block is performed by the injection of anesthetic superiorly at the glabella, midline, and laterally at the superior nasal side walls, and either

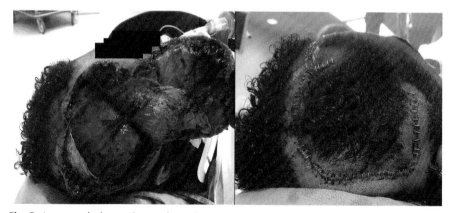

Fig. 3. Large scalp laceration and repair.

transmalar or intraorally to address the infraorbital nerves. Nasal lacerations should be repaired in layers (inner lining, cartilage, skin). The inner lining should be repaired with absorbable sutures and intranasal stenting considered during the healing process to prevent contracture and stenosis.[19] Cartilage injuries should be repaired with absorbable monofilament sutures to restore the natural contour. **Fig. 4** depicts a full thickness alar laceration and repair, which was performed in layers.

In cases of avulsion, the avulsed segment should be replaced if available. If the avulsed segment is not available, the wound can be grafted acutely, ideally within weeks of the injury, with a full-thickness or composite graft.[2] Alternatively, the wound can be allowed to granulate with a plan for delayed reconstruction.[19] Nasal injuries are susceptible to significant contracture and subsequent collapse of the cartilaginous structure, which should be considered when deciding optimal repair and timing.[2] Particular attention should be paid to meticulous closure and realignment of the wound margin in lacerations involving the alar rim. Failure to appropriately alight the alar margin can lead to alar notching and cosmetic deformity. Despite the surgeon's best efforts, healing nasal wounds can lead to cosmetic deformity and may require rhinoplasty to repair; in these cases, it is recommended to wait at least 9 to 12 months before performing rhinoplasty. For those cases where soft tissue reconstruction cannot be achieved collaboration with an anaplastologist for prosthesis is a viable option.[12]

Eyelid Lacerations

Eyelid injuries should be evaluated for underlying bony injuries, injury to the lacrimal apparatus, and evaluation of extraocular muscle injuries. The evaluation should also include inspection for retro-orbital hematoma, which may necessitate lateral canthotomy and cantholysis. Injuries to the globe or lacrimal apparatus necessitate ophthalmology consultation. The eyelid is divided anatomically into posterior lamella (tarsus and conjunctiva) and anterior lamella (skin and orbicularis oculi muscle), which should be reapproximated separately.[2] Anterior lamellar injuries do not require the reapproximation of the orbicularis oculi muscle and should not be incorporated into skin closure to prevent tethering of the eyelid.[2] Eyelid lacerations can be categorized into partial and full-thickness lacerations. Full-thickness lacerations, by definition, involve the posterior lamella in cases where periorbital edema limits examination application of

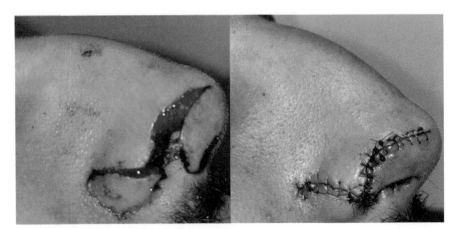

Fig. 4. Full thickness nasal laceration repair.

ice for 20 minutes can be helpful.[20] An examination should include evaluation for the involvement of the tarsus, which can be accomplished by gentle eversion of the upper and lower eyelids.[20] Failure to recognize and repair the tarsus can lead to eyelid notching, with aesthetic deformity and defects in eyelash function. Lacerations to the medial eyelid pose a risk for injury to the lacrimal system. Unrepaired injuries to the lacrimal system can lead to chronic epiphora. The puncta of the superior and inferior eyelids lie in the medial aspect of the canthi, respectively. The lacrimal drainage system runs horizontally for approximately 8 mm to join the common canaliculus, which then connects to the nasolacrimal duct.[20] Lacerations occurring medial to the punctum require the probing of the lacrimal system to assess for injury. If an injury to the canaliculus is identified, a stent should be placed, and the laceration should be closed while leaving the stent in place. Repair in the operating room should be considered, as research has shown improved outcomes.[21] Secondary repair of canalicular injuries is challenging; therefore, repair by a surgeon experienced with canalicular lacerations should occur. In cases where the injury cannot be repaired immediately, antibiotic ointment and nonadherent dressing should be applied to the laceration, or a moisture chamber may be used if the cornea is exposed.

Burn Injuries/Caustic Injuries

Patients sustaining burn or caustic injuries to the head and or neck may also be at risk for inhalation injuries. Securing the airway is a top priority. Periocular burns should prompt woods lamp examination, and if corneal abrasions are noted, ophthalmology should be consulted.[22] Injury severity will dictate treatment. Friedstat and Klein report a goal of treatment completion within 3 weeks of the injury, those not fully healed at this time point are skingrafted.[22] Facial burn wounds should first be debrided of loose blisters and debris. Wounds are then reassessed at 10 days after injury and further debridement occurs if necessary. Wounds that are not healed 21 days after the initial injury are then skin grafted.[22] Twice daily wound care is important and specific wound dressing is determined by the injury severity. Topical antibiotic ointment (such as bacitracin) should be applied to partial thickness burns, and silver sulfadiazine applied to deeper burns.[22] **Fig. 5** shows facial burn and subsequent debridement. **Fig. 6** shows the same patient at 6 months and 18 months after treatment.

Frostbite

The nasal and auricular regions are especially susceptible to frostbite and can be seriously injured. Frostbite occurs when the soft tissue freezes, causing hypoxia and tissue ischemia. Various classification schemes exist for staging injury severity but

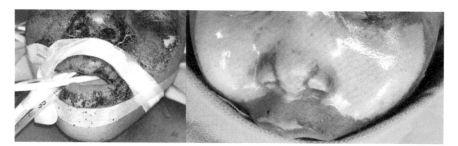

Fig. 5. Facial burn patient before and debridement.

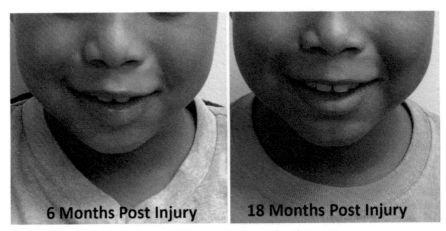

Fig. 6. Facial burn patient from **Fig. 5** at 6 and 18 months after treatment.

treatment centers around the temperature of involved tissue. For tissue that is frozen or cold active rewarming should be started.[23] Rewarming involves the application of a 40°C solution to involved tissue over 30 minutes.[24] This is a painful process and should be treated with narcotic analgesics. In addition to rapid warming and analgesics, treatment should include antibiotics.[3] Hyperbaric oxygen therapy may be considered for tissue not responsive to rapid warming.[23]

Human/Dog Bites

In cases of bites, rabies, and tetanus, immunization is recommended, and given the high incidence of wound contamination, antibiotics are also recommended.[3] Studies have shown that canine bite injuries can be closed primarily if there is no tissue loss.[3] However, there is less data regarding human bites, so delayed closure may be considered. Antibiotic treatment should ensure coverage for Pasturella multocida, which has been shown to cause nearly half of the infections after canine bites.[3] **Fig. 7** depicts a dog bite to the face and the repair.

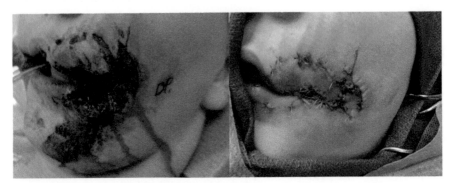

Fig. 7. Dog bite to the face before and after repair.

SUMMARY

The facial trauma surgeon will see a wide breadth of facial injuries. Optimal patient care requires the recognition of injuries that could lead to long-term complications and recognition of injuries that require subspecialty care. This can mean involving an ophthalmologist or microvascular surgeon in the trauma patient's care.

CLINICS CARE POINTS

- Recognize and repair tarsal injuries to prevent the notching of the eyelid
- Recognize cases where microvascular repair is indicated (total scalp or total auricular avulsion) and expedite transfer to a microvascular surgeon
- Canalicular injuries require stenting and should be repaired by those experienced in this repair

DISCLOSURE

The authors have no disclosures.

REFERENCES

1. Perry M, Dancey A, Mireskandari K, et al. Emergency care in facial trauma–a maxillofacial and ophthalmic perspective. Injury 2005;36(8):875–96.
2. Cho DY, Willborg BE, Lu GN. Management of traumatic soft tissue injuries of the face. Semin Plast Surg 2021;35(4):229–37.
3. Ramachandra T, Ries WR. Management of nasal and perinasal soft tissue injuries. Facial Plast Surg 2015;31(3):194–200.
4. Abubaker AO. Use of prophylactic antibiotics in preventing infection of traumatic injuries. Oral Maxillofacial Surg Clin N Am 2009;21(2):259–64, vii.
5. Gailey AD, Farquhar D, Clark JM, et al. Auricular avulsion injuries and reattachment techniques: a systematic review. Laryngoscope Investig Otolaryngol 2020;5(3):381–9.
6. Luo X, Yang J, Yang Q, et al. Classification and reconstruction of posttraumatic ear deformity. J Craniofac Surg 2012;23(3):654–7.
7. Lavasani L, Leventhal D, Constantinides M, et al. Management of acute soft tissue injury to the auricle. Facial Plast Surg 2010;26(6):445–50.
8. Steffen A, Katzbach R, Klaiber S. A comparison of ear reattachment methods: a review of 25 years since Pennington. Plast Reconstr Surg 2006;118(6):1358–64.
9. Shelley OP, Villafane O, Watson SB. Successful partial ear replantation after prolonged ischaemia time. Br J Plast Surg 2000;53(1):76–7.
10. Erdmann D, Bruno AD, Follmar KE, et al. The helical arcade: anatomic basis for survival in near-total ear avulsion. J Craniofac Surg 2009;20(1):245–8.
11. Bai H, Tollefson TT. Treatment strategies for auricular avulsions: best practice. JAMA Facial Plast Surg 2014;16(1):7–8.
12. Klimczak J, Helman S, Kadakia S, et al. Prosthetics in facial reconstruction. Craniomaxillofac Trauma Reconstr 2018;11(1):6–14.
13. Yang SH, Park H, Yoo DS, et al. Microsurgical anatomy of the facial nerve. Clin Anat 2021;34(1):90–102.
14. Greywoode JD, Ho HH, Artz GJ, et al. Management of traumatic facial nerve injuries. Facial Plast Surg 2010;26(6):511–8.

15. Lee LN, Lyford-Pike S, Boahene KD. Traumatic facial nerve injury. Otolaryngol Clin North Am 2013;46(5):825–39.
16. Sabatino F, Moskovitz JB. Facial wound management. Emerg Med Clin North Am 2013;31(2):529–38.
17. Jin Y, Hua C, Hu X, et al. Microsurgical replantation of total avulsed scalp: extending the limits. J Craniofac Surg 2017;28(3):670–4.
18. Decker JR, Dutton JM. Local anesthesia for nasal and sinus surgery. Ear Nose Throat J 2013;92(3):107–8.
19. Farrior EH, Eisler LS. Cosmetic concerns related to the posttraumatic nose without nasal obstruction. Facial Plast Surg 2015;31(3):270–9.
20. Ko AC, Satterfield KR, Korn BS, et al. Eyelid and periorbital soft tissue trauma. Facial Plast Surg Clin North Am 2017;25(4):605–16.
21. Murchison AP, Bilyk JR. Canalicular laceration repair: an analysis of variables affecting success. Ophthal Plast Reconstr Surg 2014;30(5):410–4.
22. Friedstat JS, Klein MB. Acute management of facial burns. Clin Plast Surg 2009; 36(4):653–60.
23. Sheridan RL, Goverman JM, Walker TG. Diagnosis and treatment of frostbite. N Engl J Med 2022;386(23):2213–20.
24. Osetinsky LM, Hamilton GS 3rd, Carlson ML. Sport injuries of the ear and temporal bone. Clin Sports Med 2017;36(2):315–35.

Penetrating Head and Neck Trauma

A Narrative Review of Evidence-Based Evaluation and Treatment Protocols

James M. Hamilton, MD[a,b,*], Tyler G. Chan, BS[c],
Charles E. Moore, MD[a,b]

KEYWORDS

- Head and neck trauma • Penetrating injury • No-zone framework
- Evidence-based protocols

KEY POINTS

- Penetrating injury to the head and neck accounts for a minority of trauma but significant morbidity in the US civilian population.
- The 3-zone anatomical framework has historically guided evaluation and management; however, the most current evidence-based protocols favor a no-zone approach.
- In stable patients, a thorough physical examination and noninvasive imaging should be prioritized, with surgical exploration of the head and neck reserved for certain circumstances.
- Diagnostic and management decisions should be tailored to the patient's mechanism of injury, trauma history, physical examination, experience of personnel, availability of equipment, and clinical judgment.

INTRODUCTION

Head and neck trauma poses diagnostic and management challenges due to the complexity and importance of the aerodigestive, vascular, and neurologic structures contained within.[1] Although this small anatomical region represents only 2.9% of all trauma cases in the United States, its case fatality rate is 17.36%—the highest rate of all body regions.[2] Given this mortality rate, protocols governing the evaluation,

[a] Department of Otolaryngology–Head and Neck Surgery, Emory University School of Medicine, Atlanta, GA, USA; [b] Department of Otolaryngology–Head and Neck Surgery, Grady Memorial Hospital, Atlanta, GA, USA; [c] Emory University School of Medicine, Atlanta, GA, USA
* Corresponding author. Department of Otolaryngology-Head and Neck Surgery, Emory University School of Medicine, 80 Gilmer Street, 6th Floor, Atlanta, GA 30303.
E-mail address: james.hamilton@emory.edu

Otolaryngol Clin N Am 56 (2023) 1013–1025
https://doi.org/10.1016/j.otc.2023.05.006
0030-6665/23/© 2023 Elsevier Inc. All rights reserved.

triage, and management of patients with penetrating head and neck trauma must be closely examined to optimize patient outcomes.

Penetrating neck trauma is defined as injury that pierces deep to the platysma muscle.[3] The most common mechanism worldwide is stab wounds, followed by gunshot wounds (GSWs), self-harm, road traffic accidents, and other high-velocity objects.[4] Through World War II, surgical exploration was the primary diagnostic and therapeutic modality for such injuries, likely due to the absence of informative diagnostic techniques and high morbidity associated with delayed treatment.[5] An anatomically guided classification that delineated the head and neck region into zones was introduced in 1969 to describe the location of injury and provide a framework to consider injuries to structures housed within each zone.[6,7] The current 3-zone classification evolved from this delineation and has since featured prominently in many protocols[8] (**Table 1**).

Traditionally, when evaluating hemodynamically stable patients with penetrating neck trauma, this framework has mandated surgical exploration of injuries to Zone 2, and recommended a more selective approach for the other zones due to difficult surgical access to the skull base and thoracic inlet.[8] More recently, the widespread availability of high-quality cross-sectional imaging such as computed tomography angiography (CTA) has challenged the paradigm of mandated surgical intervention.[9]

NATURE OF THE PROBLEM

Unstable patients who present with "hard" signs of vascular or aerodigestive tract injury warrant emergent surgical exploration.[10] Whether to operate on stable patients with "soft" signs, or asymptomatic patients, is less clear.[11] Problems associated with the zone-based approach include high-negative neck exploration rates in stable injuries (13%–19%), poor correlation between the wound location and internal organ injuries, and difficulty grouping multilevel injuries into one zone.[10] Routine neck exploration in hemodynamically stable patients results in longer hospitalizations and

Table 1
Historic divisions of penetrating head and neck injury into zones

Zone	Boundaries	Structures
3	Skull base to angle of mandible	Vascular: carotid arteries, jugular veins, vertebral arteries Pulmonary: pharynx Gastrointestinal: N/A Neurologic: spinal cord, cranial nerves, sympathetic chain ganglia Other: salivary glands
2	Angle of mandible to cricoid cartilage	Vascular: internal/external carotid arteries Pulmonary: pharynx, larynx Gastrointestinal: esophagus Neurologic: spinal cord, vagus nerve, recurrent laryngeal nerve Other: N/A
1	Cricoid cartilage to clavicles	Vascular: subclavian artery/vein, vertebral artery/vein, carotid arteries, jugular veins Pulmonary: trachea, lungs Gastrointestinal: esophagus Neurologic: spinal cord, vagus nerve Other: thoracic duct, thyroid gland

Adapted from Weale R, Madsen A, Kong V, Clarke D. (2019). The management of penetrating neck injury. Trauma, 21(2), 85-93.

increased rates of complications (surgical site infections, sepsis, and so forth).[12] Yet there are no international consensus guidelines regarding decisions to operate.

With the advent of CTA, most current evidence-based studies support a shift away from zone-based algorithms toward less-invasive diagnostic procedures and selective surgery after consideration of the patient's status.[1,4,9-11,13-15] This is termed the "no-zone" approach. The goal of this review is to outline current evidence-based practices for evaluation and management of penetrating head and neck trauma.

EVALUATION

Signs of injury in penetrating neck trauma can be classified as "hard" or "soft" based on severity (**Table 2**). Patients may also be asymptomatic. Physical examination is indicated in all patients with penetrating wounds to the head or neck, due to its high sensitivity for injury detection[16,17] and the high risk of decompensating from asphyxiation and exsanguination.[12,18] Initial evaluation involves resuscitation according to advanced trauma life-support principles. A patent airway is the first priority. If airway compromise is suspected, rapid-sequence intubation is indicated when anatomic structures of the head and neck are preserved and airway anatomy can be clearly visualized. Intubation should occur only with clear visualization,[4,19,20] to avoid forcing air into injured tissue planes or further distorting airway anatomy.[4,21,22] Fiberoptic laryngoscopy can help achieve visualization. If intubation fails, or is precluded by disfiguring facial injuries, either immediate emergent tracheotomy or cricothyrotomy is

Table 2
Hard" and "Soft" signs of head and neck injury

Hard Signs	Soft Signs
Vascular	• Stable hematoma
• Refractory shock	• Hoarseness
• Rapidly expanding hematoma	• Dysphagia
• Uncontrolled hemorrhage	• Mild subcutaneous emphysema
• Absent pulse	• Mild hematemesis/hemoptysis
• Audible bruit or palpable thrill	• Dysphonia
Respiratory	• Odynophagia
• Airway compromise	• Chest pain
• Wound bubbling	
• Subcutaneous emphysema	
• Stridor/hoarseness	
• Massive hemoptysis	
• Air sucking in and out	
• Impaired speech	
• Cyanosis	
• Respiratory distress	
• Air bubbling from wound site	
Esophageal	
• Severe dysphagia	
• Significant hematemesis	
Neurologic	
• Neurological deficits	

The presence of any "hard" sign is an indication for surgical exploration of penetrating head and neck trauma.
Adapted from Chandrananth, M. L., Zhang, A., Voutier, C. R., Skandarajah, A., Thomson, B. N. J., Shakerian, R., & Read, D. J. (2021). 'No zone' approach to the management of stable penetrating neck injuries: a systematic review. ANZ journal of surgery, 91(6), 1083–1090.

indicated. Once the airway is secured, attention should turn to hemodynamics and establishing intravenous access before surgical intervention. Direct laryngoscopy, bronchoscopy, or esophagoscopy should be used as necessary to further identify injuries across systems and guide management.[23]

CONSIDERATIONS

The management of patients who present with soft signs or no symptoms is less clear. A benign-appearing entry site can belie the severity of injury because the depth and trajectory of penetration are hidden.[21] The degree of tissue damage depends on the kinetic energy transferred from the penetrating object to the neck tissue,[24] which in turn depends on the mass and velocity of the missile.[18] The energy of a projectile can radiate beyond the perforation site, creating a cavity up to 30 times its size.[25] Thus, penetrating injuries to the head and neck are considered life-threatening until proven otherwise.[21,22]

Injuries from knives or thrown objects generally cause less damage than ballistic injuries, which are more difficult to assess.[26] GSWs can be divided into low-velocity and high-velocity injuries. Small-caliber handguns cause less collateral tissue damage along the projectile path than high-powered rifles or shotguns, which produce a large

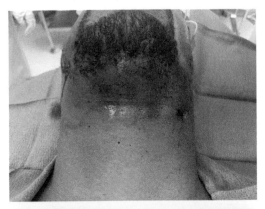

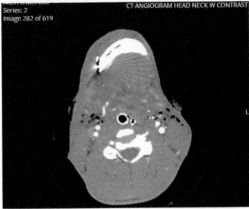

CT ANGIOGRAM HEAD NECK W CONTRAST
Series: 2
Image 282 of 619

Fig. 1. A 31-year-old man with a GSW to left neck zone II with CTA showing no vascular injury. Given the lack of hard signs of vascular and respiratory injury and stable vital signs, neck exploration was avoided and patient underwent elective repair of mandible fracture on hospital day 2.

concussive wave that can disrupt tissue, rupture blood vessels and nerves, and fracture bones despite their distance from the permanent cavity of the missile (**Fig. 1**).[27] Structures distant from the entry site must also be evaluated. Impaled objects should not be removed until the extent of injury can be elucidated, and wounds should not be blindly probed, to avoid iatrogenic injury.[21,24] Knowledge of the mechanism of injury is useful in predicting damage and crucial for proper management.[25]

THE DECISION TO OPERATE

Three anatomic zones have been used to categorize wounds by entry location and to guide treatment (see **Table 1**).[4,7,8,25] Using this algorithm, a penetrating wound of Zone 2 in stable patients is an indication for surgical exploration, and patients with a Zone 1 or 3 injury should undergo endoscopy and angiography due to more difficult surgical access to these regions.[28] There has been unclear benefit of civilian adoption of mandatory surgical intervention as negative neck exploration rates are reported as high as 56%.[10] These highly invasive, labor-intensive procedures also increase complication rates and prolong hospitalization.[27,29–31] Furthermore, location of entry and injury often do not correlate with underlying structures.[32] Thus, management based solely on zones can easily result in inappropriate management decisions.

  Historically, various imaging modalities have been used, including 4-vessel digital subtraction angiography,[33] color Doppler,[34] and magnetic resonance angiography. Universal application has been impractical, however, due to risk of complications, operator dependency, and magnetic interaction with possible impaled objects, respectively. More recently, spiral multidirectory CTA has become the favored diagnostic imaging tool due to its high-quality images, speed, and minimally invasive nature. With its low cost and widespread availability in modern trauma centers, it has become an integral to the selective, symptom-based approach[9] that has greatly simplified the management of penetrating neck trauma while reducing the number of missed injuries and negative neck exploration rates.[10]

No-Zone Systems-Based Management

Treatment using the no-zone approach is based on the classification of symptoms that may reflect damage to the major organ systems.

Vascular

Up to 25% of penetrating head and neck injuries result in vascular trauma, including intimal flap, arteriovenous fistula, pseudoaneurysm, and rupture. Mortality rate approaches 50%.[14,24,35,36] The mechanism of death is often exsanguination.[37] Therefore, the presence of hard signs of vascular head and neck trauma warrants surgical exploration.[4] The most common vascular injury from penetrating neck trauma is to the common carotid artery in Zone 2. Damage to the vertebral arteries is rare but possible, with risk factors for stroke and mortality more closely associated with medical history and associated injuries than with treatment decisions.[38,39] Interruption of vertebral artery blood flow is well tolerated due to excellent posterior circulation, and ligation or embolization is the treatment of choice in most injuries requiring intervention.[6,38] Bilateral internal jugular vein injury warrants careful management due to the potential for facial and cerebral edema.[40]

Laryngotracheal

Injury of the larynx and trachea is uncommon in penetrating head and neck trauma but can incur substantial morbidity and mortality if not detected and addressed promptly.[41,42] Once the airway is secure, attention can turn to the location and extent of injury. In stable patients, chest radiograph can help identify tracheal deviations or bone fractures. Vocal cord function should be assessed with flexible laryngoscopy. Direct laryngoscopy or rigid bronchoscopy may be used to localize injury. Exposed or structurally compromised cartilage must be addressed surgically to maintain airway patency and long-term preservation of phonation. Voice quality and airway patency may be improved when surgery is performed within 24 hours.[43]

Noninvasive procedures include head-of-bed elevation and antiemetics for reflux precautions, serial physical examination to assess for progressive airway compromise from occult hematoma, and steroids to control edema.

Pharyngoesophageal

The reported incidence of injuries to the pharynx and esophagus is under 10%.[41] Although most recommend a conservative approach to surgical intervention,[42,44] delayed recognition and treatment of pharyngoesophageal injury leads to increased morbidity and mortality due to leakage of digestive fluids through occult injuries producing necrotic inflammatory responses.[45,46] Mortality rates up to 20% have been reported.[47,48] Others cite high false-negative rates and advocate for wide, early use of esophagography and rigid esophagoscopy.[49,50]

Neurologic. Neurologic structures at risk of involvement include the spinal cord, cranial nerves, the sympathetic chain, peripheral nerve roots, and the brachial plexus.[4] Spinal cord injuries represent less than 1% of penetrating neck injuries; however, their sequelae can be devastating.[26] Spinal cord transection above C5 will produce paraplegia and can cause respiratory distress from disrupted innervation to the diaphragm. Spinal cord lesions can also elicit neurogenic shock from unopposed parasympathetic and vagal tone; therefore, signs of hypotension or bradycardia should be carefully monitored.[21] Placement of a cervical collar is not routinely recommended in the absence of neurological signs as unnecessary immobilization of the cervical spine may actually hinder management by obscuring airway visualization, hiding injuries, and obstructing assessment of neck wounds.[4]

A comprehensive neurologic examination is warranted as part of the initial survey and should be documented on all patients to identify the extent and timing of any deficit.[21] Injury to the facial nerve can result in impaired eyelid closure, oral incompetence, and mastication difficulty. Vagal nerve injury can impair vocal cord mobility, leading to dysphonia, dysphagia, aspiration, and airway compromise. Patients with penetrating neck injuries are also at risk of cerebrovascular insults from temporary or prolonged ischemia or released emboli from compromised vertebral or carotid arteries.

Penetrating trauma of the face

Penetrating facial trauma presents its own diagnostic and management challenges. The National Trauma Data Bank reports a case fatality rate of 14.9%.[2] GSWs are most common in the United States[51] and can be categorized as nonpenetrating (abrasion of the skin), penetrating (the projectile enters but does not exit the face), perforating (presence of entry and exit points), or avulsive (entry and exit with substantial tissue loss).[52] The primary objective is to sustain life, followed by restoration of facial form and function. Once patients have been stabilized and imaging obtained, repair and reconstruction are implemented according to the reconstructive ladder.

The rate of surgical intervention after facial GSWs ranges from 38% to 100%,[53] with few guidelines regarding the decision to operate.[51,53,54] A study of patients with isolated facial GSWs showed an association between location and surgical intervention: injuries to the lower face (below the occlusal plane to the angle of the mandible) required surgical intervention more often (87.2%) than those to the upper (60%;

supraorbital rim to infraorbital rim) or middle face (29.6%; infraorbital rim to occlusal plane).[55] Another study categorized facial GSWs by location of injury: temporal, frontal, intraoral, submental, or neck.[56] Mortality was 82% among patients with temporal bone injury versus 14% for submental injury, suggesting that proximity of entry wounds to the cranial cavity is predictive of mortality.

Another study of lower face injuries emphasized the timing of treatment.[51] The authors divided time after admission into emergency (day of presentation), immediate surgery (within 72 hours), delayed surgery (72 hours to 2 weeks), and secondary intervention (after 2 weeks) phases and recommended addressing fractures within 72 hours for best results, with exceptions for concomitant life-threatening or cranial injuries mandating earlier attention. They also recommended delayed osseous reconstruction to allow adequate time for soft-tissue closure. Others advocate delay to allow edema to resolve, facilitating better assessment of facial contours and optimal esthetic outcomes after reconstruction.[57,58] Nonetheless, immediate reconstruction confers benefits such as reductions in tissue fibrosis, length of hospitalization, and periods of suboptimal esthetic appearance.

Current Evidence

Growing evidence supports giving more emphasis to patients' signs, symptoms, and imaging in dictating investigation and management.[10] Multiple studies of patients undergoing CTA, including several prospective studies, reported sensitivity of 93.9% to 100% and specificity of 93.5% to 97.5% in detecting all vascular and aerodigestive injuries regardless of ultimate treatment modality.[10,11,13,15,52,59]

Patients with Hard Signs

The literature shows consensus in advocating for mandatory surgical exploration in patients who present with hard signs[52,59,60] (**Fig. 2**), although some evidence suggest that preoperative CTA is reasonable (**Fig. 1**). A recent study identified no significant difference in missed injuries between CTA and surgical exploration in patients with Zone 2 injuries presenting with hard signs, with rates of negative neck exploration of 0% in the CTA group versus 36% in the operative group.[15] In another study of patients with hard signs who underwent CTA due to hemodynamic stability, 61.5% underwent surgery, allowing 38.5% to avoid neck exploration.[13] Another study reported a decrease in negative neck exploration rate from of 23% to 15% with use of CTA among stable patients with hard signs.[61] All studies showed decreased rates of negative neck exploration with no consequent complications, missed injuries, or mortality.[13,15,61] Thus, preoperative CTA in patients presenting with hard signs may be warranted if the patient can be stabilized (see **Fig. 1**).

Patients with Soft Signs

A prospective, single-center cohort study evaluated the benefit of CTA screening in the initial evaluation of patients with penetrating neck injuries who were symptomatic with soft signs.[52] Of these, 17.7% required surgery, meaning 82.3% avoided unnecessary neck exploration. Another study reported a negative neck exploration rate of 0% for patients who underwent CTA, with a rate of 48% reported for 27 non-CTA patients.[62] Other reports similarly found that the use of CTA led to the avoidance of negative neck exploration in 51.7% to 97.7% of patients with soft signs.[10,61,63,64] These studies support management with CTA and close observation, showing very few missed injuries or complications in patients with soft signs.

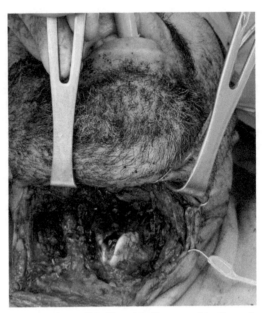

Fig. 2. A 29-year-old man with a self-inflicted knife wound to the anterior neck in zone II underwent neck exploration due to active hemorrhage, respiratory distress and stridor, and exposed laryngeal cartilage. Bilateral carotid arteries were found to be intact but a transection of the thyro-hyoid membrane was identified with open communication of the lumen of the hypopharynx and larynx. Wound was evaluated with intraop direct laryngoscopy, flexible esophagoscopy, and bronchoscopy. Injury was repaired primarily with mucosal inverting stitches and bolstered with a rotational muscle flap using strap muscles.

Patients with No Signs

For asymptomatic patients, diagnosis and management modalities are also unclear. Although mandatory neck exploration is less advised, the benefit of CTA is less established. Many studies support the use of thorough physical examination. Several studies have shown no missed injuries reported no further complications with serial physical examinations and close observation.[10,59] Another study reported that among 99 asymptomatic patients, 3 revealed positive CTA findings, with none resulting in delayed complications or requiring surgery.[63] However, one study found that 2 of 41 asymptomatic patients had injury (tracheal puncture and pseudoaneurysm) after CTA,[52] and another showed vascular injury in 5% of asymptomatic patients who underwent CTA based on the surgeon's discretion; these were all GSWs.[13] Therefore, CTA may not be indicated in most asymptomatic patients, perhaps except for those with GSWs.

Potential Drawbacks

Despite the benefits of CTA, occult injuries have been discovered on surgical exploration not identified on CTA.[65,66] Historically, the morbidity and mortality of missed esophageal injuries was a strong driver of mandatory surgical exploration.[3] One study indicated the sensitivity of CTA in detecting pharyngoesophageal injuries to be as low as 53%.[47] A punctured airway or perforated esophagus is less likely to be detected by

CTA. Thus, barium swallow, esophagoscopy, bronchoscopy, or fluoroscopy added to CTA warrants consideration.[11]

Finally, the false-positive rate of CTA should not be ignored. One study showed 5 false-positive diagnoses of aerodigestive tract injuries that resulted in 2 negative neck explorations.[52] Another showed a false-positive CTA rate of 14.8%.[13] A nonnegligible risk of detecting clinically insignificant injuries might drive further workup or exploration when none is therapeutically necessary. Additionally, the quality of CTA imaging is occasionally hampered by streak artifacts, and IV contrast is contraindicated in some patients.[14,60] Increased radiation burden should also be considered.[59] Thus regardless of CTA findings, a high index of suspicion should be maintained and serial physical examinations performed in all patients with penetrating head and neck trauma to prevent missed injuries.

SUMMARY

Although penetrating trauma to the head and neck is relatively uncommon, the risks of untreated or unrecognized sequelae are potentially life-threatening. The current evidence-based literature favors noninvasive imaging over mandatory surgical exploration, regardless of zone of injury. Imaging triage accomplishes safe, noninvasive evaluation of head and neck structures to rule in or out injury warranting surgical intervention. Invasive algorithms should be replaced with a new standard of care: evidence-based screening strategies comprising physical examination and CTA. Protocols and guidelines continue to evolve as novel diagnostic and therapeutic techniques are introduced to provide optimal outcomes for patients with penetrating injury of the head and neck.

CLINICS CARE POINTS

- High-quality images, speed, and minimally invasive nature have mad spiral multidirectory CTA the favored diagnostic imaging tool due for penetrating trauma to the head and neck. With its low cost and widespread availability in modern trauma centers, it has become an integral to the selective, symptom-based approach that has greatly simplified the management of penetrating neck trauma while reducing the number of missed injuries and negative neck exploration rates.

- Growing evidence supports giving more emphasis to patients' signs, symptoms, and imaging in dictating investigation and management..

- The literature shows consensus for mandatory surgical exploration in patients who present with hard signs of vascular or aerodigestive tract injury, although some evidence suggests that preoperative CTA may be warranted if the patient can be stabilized.

- In the patient with soft signs, the literature supports management with CTA and close observation, showing very few missed injuries or complications in patients with soft signs.

- CTA may not be indicated in most asymptomatic patients, perhaps except for those with GSWs.

- Regardless of CTA findings, a high index of suspicion should be maintained, and serial physical examinations performed in all patients with penetrating head and neck trauma to prevent missed injuries.

DISCLOSURE

The authors have no funding, financial relationships, or conflicts of interest to disclose.

REFERENCES

1. Shiroff AM, Gale SC, Martin ND, et al. Penetrating Neck Trauma: A Review of Management Strategies and Discussion of the 'No Zone' Approach. Am Surg 2013;79:23–9.
2. National Trauma Data bank 2016 Annual Report. American College of Surgeons; 2016.
3. Fogelman MJ, Stewart RD. Penetrating wounds of the neck. Am J Surg 1956; 91(4):581–96.
4. Nowicki JL, Stew B, Ooi E. Penetrating neck injuries: a guide to evaluation and management. Ann R Coll Surg Engl 2018;100(1):6–11.
5. Miller RH, Duplechain JK. Penetrating wounds of the neck. Otolaryngol Clin North Am 1991;24(1):15–29.
6. Kesser BW, Chance E, Kleiner D, et al. Contemporary management of penetrating neck trauma. Am Surg 2009;75(1):1–10.
7. Monson DO, Saletta JD, Freeark RJ. Carotid vertebral trauma. J Trauma 1969; 9(12):987–99.
8. Roon AJ, Christensen N. Evaluation and treatment of penetrating cervical injuries. J Trauma 1979;19(6):391–7.
9. Chandrananth ML, Zhang A, Voutier CR, et al. 'No zone' approach to the management of stable penetrating neck injuries: a systematic review. ANZ J Surg 2021; 91(6):1083–90.
10. Prichayudh S, Choadrachata-anun J, Sriussadaporn S, et al. Selective management of penetrating neck injuries using "no zone" approach. Injury 2015;46(9): 1720–5.
11. Amico F, Bendinelli C, Balogh ZJ. Penetrating neck trauma: No zone, no problem? ANZ J Surg 2021;91(6):1051–2.
12. Ko JW, Gong SC, Kim MJ, et al. The efficacy of the "no zone" approach for the assessment of traumatic neck injury: a case-control study. Ann Surg Treat Res 2020;99(6):352–61.
13. Madsen AS, Kong VY, Oosthuizen GV, et al. Computed Tomography Angiography is the Definitive Vascular Imaging Modality for Penetrating Neck Injury: A South African Experience. Scand J Surg 2018;107(1):23–30.
14. Kee-Sampson JW, Gopireddy DR, Vulasala SSR, et al. Role of imaging in penetrating vascular injuries of the craniocervical region. J Clin Imaging Sci 2022; 12:63.
15. Schroll R, Fontenot T, Lipcsey M, et al. Role of computed tomography angiography in the management of Zone II penetrating neck trauma in patients with clinical hard signs. J Trauma Acute Care Surg 2015;79(6):943–50 [discussion: 950].
16. Eddy VA. Is routine arteriography mandatory for penetrating injury to zone 1 of the neck? Zone 1 Penetrating Neck Injury Study Group. J Trauma 2000;48(2):208–13 [discussion: 213–4].
17. Azuaje RE, Jacobson LE, Glover J, et al. Reliability of physical examination as a predictor of vascular injury after penetrating neck trauma. Am Surg 2003;69(9): 804–7.
18. Siau RT, Moore A, Ahmed T, et al. Management of penetrating neck injuries at a London trauma centre. Eur Arch Oto-Rhino-Laryngol 2013;270(7):2123–8.
19. Tallon JM, Ahmed JM, Sealy B. Airway management in penetrating neck trauma at a Canadian tertiary trauma centre. Cjem 2007;9(2):101–4.
20. Youssef N, Raymer KE. Airway management of an open penetrating neck injury. Cjem 2015;17(1):89–93.

21. Kesser BW, Chance E, Kleiner D, et al. Article Commentary: Contemporary Management of Penetrating Neck Trauma. Am Surg 2009;75(1):1–10.
22. Kendall JL, Anglin D, Demetriades D. Penetrating neck trauma. Emerg Med Clin North Am 1998;16(1):85–105.
23. Paul W, Flint BH, Lund V, et al. Cummings otolaryngology head and neck surgery. Elsevier; 2020.
24. Rhee P, Kuncir EJ, Johnson L, et al. Cervical spine injury is highly dependent on the mechanism of injury following blunt and penetrating assault. J Trauma 2006; 61(5):1166–70.
25. Asensio JA, Valenziano CP, Falcone RE, et al. Management of penetrating neck injuries. The controversy surrounding zone II injuries. Surg Clin North Am 1991; 71(2):267–96.
26. Saletta JD, Lowe RJ, Lim LT, et al. Penetrating trauma of the neck. J Trauma 1976; 16(7):579–87.
27. Demetriades D, Salim A, Brown C, et al. Neck injuries. Curr Probl Surg 2007; 44(1):13–85.
28. Golueke PJ, Goldstein AS, Sclafani SJ, et al. Routine versus selective exploration of penetrating neck injuries: a randomized prospective study. J Trauma 1984; 24(12):1010–4.
29. Obeid FN, Haddad GS, Horst HM, et al. A critical reappraisal of a mandatory exploration policy for penetrating wounds of the neck. Surg Gynecol Obstet 1985;160(6):517–22.
30. Meyer JP, Barrett JA, Schuler JJ, et al. Mandatory vs selective exploration for penetrating neck trauma. A prospective assessment. Arch Surg 1987;122(5): 592–7.
31. Ashworth C, Williams LF, Byrne JJ. Penetrating wounds of the neck: Re-emphasis of the need for prompt exploration. Am J Surg 1971;121(4):387–91.
32. Low GM, Inaba K, Chouliaras K, et al. The use of the anatomic 'zones' of the neck in the assessment of penetrating neck injury. Am Surg 2014;80(10):970–4.
33. Stuhlfaut JW, Barest G, Sakai O, et al. Impact of MDCT angiography on the use of catheter angiography for the assessment of cervical arterial injury after blunt or penetrating trauma. AJR Am J Roentgenol 2005;185(4):1063–8.
34. Montalvo BM, LeBlang SD, Nuñez DB Jr, et al. Color Doppler sonography in penetrating injuries of the neck. AJNR Am J Neuroradiol 1996;17(5):943–51.
35. Stone HH, Callahan GS. SOFT TISSUE INJURIES OF THE NECK. Surg Gynecol Obstet 1963;117:745–52.
36. Saito N, Hito R, Burke PA, et al. Imaging of penetrating injuries of the head and neck:current practice at a level I trauma center in the United States. Keio J Med 2014;63(2):23–33.
37. Hong S, Klem C. Hemorrhage management and vascular control. Textbooks of military medicine otolaryngology/head and neck surgery combat casualty care in Operation Iraqi Freedom and Operation Enduring Freedom Fort Sam Houston (TX). Department of Defense (DOD), The Borden Institute; 2015.
38. Reid JD, Weigelt JA. Forty-three cases of vertebral artery trauma. J Trauma 1988; 28(7):1007–12.
39. Schellenberg M, Owattanapanich N, Cowan S, et al. Penetrating injuries to the vertebral artery: interventions and outcomes from US Trauma Centers. Eur J Trauma Emerg Surg 2022;48(1):481–8.
40. McGovern PJ Jr, Swan KG. Management of bilateral internal jugular venous injuries. Injury 1985;16(4):259–60.

41. Vassiliu P, Baker J, Henderson S, et al. Aerodigestive injuries of the neck. Am Surg 2001;67(1):75–9.
42. Demetriades D, Velmahos GG, Asensio JA. Cervical pharyngoesophageal and laryngotracheal injuries. World J Surg 2001;25(8):1044–8.
43. Bhojani RA, Rosenbaum DH, Dikmen E, et al. Contemporary assessment of laryngotracheal trauma. J Thorac Cardiovasc Surg 2005;130(2):426–32.
44. Madiba TE, Muckart DJ. Penetrating injuries to the cervical oesophagus: is routine exploration mandatory? Ann R Coll Surg Engl 2003;85(3):162–6.
45. Velmahos GC, Souter I, Degiannis E, et al. Selective surgical management in penetrating neck injuries. Can J Surg 1994;37(6):487–91.
46. Armstrong WB, Detar TR, Stanley RB. Diagnosis and management of external penetrating cervical esophageal injuries. Ann Otol Rhinol Laryngol 1994;103(11):863–71.
47. Bryant AS, Cerfolio RJ. Esophageal Trauma. Thorac Surg Clin 2007;17(1):63–72.
48. Mahmoodie M, Sanei B, Moazeni-Bistgani M, et al. Penetrating neck trauma: review of 192 cases. Arch Trauma Res 2012;1(1):14–8.
49. Weigelt JA, Thal ER, Snyder WH 3rd, et al. Diagnosis of penetrating cervical esophageal injuries. Am J Surg 1987;154(6):619–22.
50. Biffl WL, Moore EE, Rehse DH, et al. Selective management of penetrating neck trauma based on cervical level of injury. Am J Surg 1997;174(6):678–82.
51. Norris O, Mehra P, Salama A. Maxillofacial Gunshot Injuries at an Urban Level I Trauma Center—10-Year Analysis. J Oral Maxillofac Surg 2015;73(8):1532–9.
52. Demetriades D, Chahwan S, Gomez H, et al. Initial evaluation and management of gunshot wounds to the face. J Trauma 1998;45(1):39–41.
53. Chen AY, Stewart MG, Raup G. Penetrating injuries of the face. Otolaryngol Head Neck Surg 1996;115(5):464–70.
54. Qaisi M, Martin S, Al Azzawi T, et al. Is Maxillofacial Gunshot Wound Location Associated With Operative Intervention? J Oral Maxillofac Surg 2023;81(4):434–40.
55. Murphy JA, Lee MT, Liu X, et al. Factors affecting survival following self-inflicted head and neck gunshot wounds: a single-centre retrospective review. Int J Oral Maxillofac Surg 2016;45(4):513–6.
56. Peleg M, Sawatari Y. Management of gunshot wounds to the mandible. J Craniofac Surg 2010;21(4):1252–6.
57. Ueeck BA. Penetrating Injuries to the Face: Delayed Versus Primary Treatment—Considerations for Delayed Treatment. J Oral Maxillofac Surg 2007;65(6):1209–14.
58. Inaba K, Munera F, McKenney M, et al. Prospective evaluation of screening multislice helical computed tomographic angiography in the initial evaluation of penetrating neck injuries. J Trauma 2006;61(1):144–9.
59. Inaba K, Branco BC, Menaker J, et al. Evaluation of multidetector computed tomography for penetrating neck injury: a prospective multicenter study. J Trauma Acute Care Surg 2012;72(3):576–83 [discussion 583–4; quiz: 803–4].
60. Munera F, Danton G, Rivas LA, et al. Multidetector row computed tomography in the management of penetrating neck injuries. Semin Ultrasound CT MR 2009;30(3):195–204.
61. Borsetto D, Fussey J, Mavuti J, et al. Penetrating neck trauma: radiological predictors of vascular injury. Eur Arch Oto-Rhino-Laryngol 2019;276(9):2541–7.
62. Osborn TM, Bell RB, Qaisi W, et al. Computed tomographic angiography as an aid to clinical decision making in the selective management of penetrating

injuries to the neck: a reduction in the need for operative exploration. J Trauma 2008;64(6):1466–71.

63. Ibraheem K, Khan M, Rhee P, et al. "No zone" approach in penetrating neck trauma reduces unnecessary computed tomography angiography and negative explorations. J Surg Res 2018;221:113–20.

64. Hundersmarck D, Reinders Folmer E, de Borst GJ, et al. Penetrating Neck Injury in Two Dutch Level 1 Trauma Centres: the Non-Existent Problem. Eur J Vasc Endovasc Surg 2019;58(3):455–62.

65. Bhatt NR, McMonagle M. Penetrating neck injury from a screwdriver: can the No Zone approach be applied to Zone I injuries? BMJ Case Rep 2015;2015.

66. Tisherman SA, Bokhari F, Collier B, et al. Clinical practice guideline: penetrating zone II neck trauma. J Trauma 2008;64(5):1392–405.

Traumatic Injuries of the Parotid Gland and Duct

James Cochran, MD[a], Jennifer Gottfried, BS[b],
Natalya Chernichenko, MD[a,c], Rohan R. Walvekar, MD[d],
Sydney C. Butts, MD[a,c],*

KEYWORDS

- Parotid duct repair • Salivary fistula • Sialocele • Botulinum toxin

KEY POINTS

- Parotid duct injuries must be ruled out in patients with penetrating cheek trauma. Missed injuries result in significant patient morbidity.
- Successful duct repair requires microvascular reconstructive techniques.
- Sialendoscopy and botulinum toxin have an important role in the diagnosis and treatment of parotid trauma.

 Video content accompanies this article at http://www.oto.theclinics.com.

INTRODUCTION

Parotid gland (PG) injuries are rare with few studies conducted studying their incidence.[1] The primary cause of PG injury is penetrating trauma in the cheek region. Secondary causes include blunt trauma and iatrogenic injury.[2,3] Traumatic injuries of the PG and parotid duct (PD) typically occur in men aged between 25 and 35 years, with male incidences of 2 to 8 times that of women.[1,2,4,5]

Early recognition and treatment of PD injuries is essential because delays in diagnosis result in late complications. Several case series have demonstrated the natural history of untreated PD injuries by reporting the complications that developed.[1,2,6] The majority of patients in these series consistently returned for care of a sialocele or fistula

---

[a] Department of Otolaryngology, SUNY Downstate Health Sciences University, 450 Clarkson Avenue, Box 126, Brooklyn, NY 11203, USA; [b] SUNY Downstate Health Sciences University-College of Medicine, 450 Clarkson Avenue, Brooklyn, NY 11203, USA; [c] Department of Otolaryngology-Kings County Hospital Center, 451 Clarkson Avenue, Brooklyn, NY 11203, USA; [d] Department of Otolaryngology–Head and Neck Surgery, Louisiana State University Health Sciences Center, 533 Bolivar Street, Suite 566, New Orleans, LA 70112, USA
* Corresponding author.
E-mail address: sydney.butts@downstate.edu

Otolaryngol Clin N Am 56 (2023) 1027–1038
https://doi.org/10.1016/j.otc.2023.05.007
0030-6665/23/© 2023 Elsevier Inc. All rights reserved.

within days to weeks of the untreated PD injury—53% in one series—that resulted in weeks of treatment to address the complication.[1]

The PG lies posterior to the masseter muscle, overlying the ramus of the mandible, and is covered by the investing layer of deep cervical fascia. The parotid region includes the facial nerve, retromandibular vein, and branches of the external carotid artery, all of which are vulnerable to injury from trauma to this area. Running in close proximity to the PD is the transverse facial artery and the buccal branch of the facial nerve—the most commonly injured branch in PG/PD injury.[4,7] Reports indicate a high-positive predictive value for an associated facial nerve injury in the setting of PG or duct injuries with findings of 55% of PD injuries presenting with facial nerve injuries.[5]

The diameter of the PD varies along its 5 to 7 cm length, with a maximum diameter reported of 2.3 mm.[8–10] The PD originates at the anterior-superior region of the gland and runs along the masseter muscle to pierce the buccinator muscle entering the oral cavity opposite the second maxillary molar (**Fig. 1**). The PD course can be approximated by a line, which connects the tragus to the midportion of the upper lip (see **Fig. 1**).[3,11] Van Sickles' classification of PD injuries remains the most frequently cited (**Fig. 2**). Region A includes the proximal part of the duct where it exits from the gland to the posterior border of the masseter muscle; region B is the longest segment, running superficial to the masseter muscle and the most frequent site of injury; (**Fig. 3**) and region C is the distal duct beyond the anterior border of the masseter muscle.[12]

Patient Evaluation and Early Management

The initial survey of all trauma patients should follow Advanced Trauma Life Support protocols.[13] The mechanism and timing of presentation will provide key information

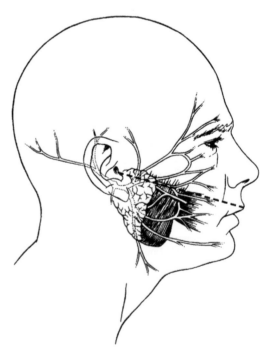

Fig. 1. The PD Line. A landmark for the PD is a line connecting the tragus to the philtrum of the upper lip. (*From* Steinberg MJ, Herrera AF. Management of parotid duct injuries. Oral Surg Oral Med Oral Pathol Oral Radiol Endod. 2005;99(2), with permission.)

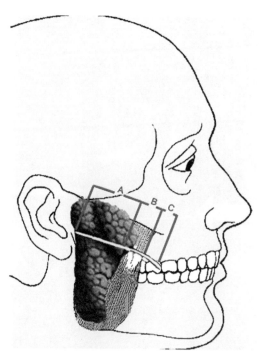

Fig. 2. Injury classification. The Van Sickles classification of PD injury divides the duct into 3 regions: Region A is the most proximal portion of duct; Region B runs superficial to the masseter muscle; and region C is the duct distal to the anterior border of the masseter muscle. (*From* Lazaridou M, Iliopoulos C, Antoniades K, Tilaveridis I, Dimitrakopoulos I, Lazaridis N. Salivary gland trauma: a review of diagnosis and treatment. *Craniomaxillofac Trauma Reconstr.* 2012;5(4):189-196., with permission.)

about the severity of the soft tissue injury and likelihood of associated injuries. Initial wound management may require control of brisk bleeding. Packing wounds and tying vessels is preferred to blind clamping until operative control is possible.[14] The examination must document baseline facial nerve function before injection of local anesthetic or administration of sedation. Information from witnesses or emergency personnel contributes to the history and examination for patients that are unresponsive. CT scan imaging with or without CT angiography should be ordered when wound hemorrhage suggests a major vascular injury, or when there are coexisting craniomaxillofacial injuries.

If time and wound conditions allow, bedside assessment of PD integrity should be attempted. Saliva pooling in the wound bed with massage of the PG suggests discontinuity of the PD. A lacrimal probe or angiocatheter can be used to cannulate the PD papilla intraorally; visualization of the probe in the wound suggests ductal injury (**Fig. 4**). Once the patient is stabilized, empiric antibiotics to cover gram-positive and oral flora and appropriate tetanus prophylaxis should be administered in preparation for operative wound exploration.

When an injury of the PG or PD is suspected, repair should be performed within 24 hours of injury.[4,15–18] Although the management of facial nerve injury is beyond the scope of this article, associated nerve transection will require simultaneous reconstruction (**Fig. 3**). Facial nerve injuries, should be explored and repaired within 72 hours, the window within which distal cut branches can be identified by nerve stimulation.[19]

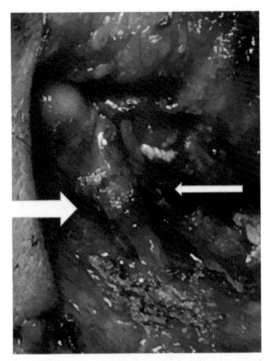

Fig. 3. PD and Facial nerve. The buccal branch of the facial nerve runs in close proximity to the PD. In this Zone B parotid duct injury, the buccal branch of the facial nerve was also transected. Both structures were repaired. The repaired PD (*wide arrow*) is shown running superior to the repaired buccal branch (*thin arrow*).

Operative Repair of Parotid Gland and Parotid Duct Injuries

The goals of management of blunt or penetrating cheek injuries are to determine the extent of PG or PD injuries if present. In some instances, injuries will be limited to the parotid parenchyma and fascia with no ductal injuries but these must also be meticulously addressed to avoid later complications.

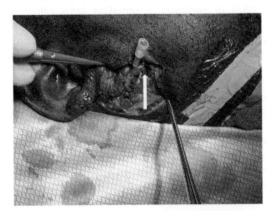

Fig. 4. Complex PD injury. A thin lacrimal probe (*arrow*) was used to cannulate the papilla of Stensen duct exiting the distal stump. The duct injury resulted in numerous lacerations along the path with a middle segment cannulated by the angiocath.

Preoperative Preparation: Informed Consent Discussion

Extensive soft tissue injuries should be anticipated, and this should organize the consent discussion had with all patients before wound exploration. The planned procedure should include the following components.

1. *Wound exploration and debridement* (especially in instances of possible retained foreign material): The consent conversation must also indicate the possibility of nerve injury as a result of wound exploration.
2. *Primary repair of the PD*: This is the gold standard when both ends are identified, and repair can be accomplished in a tension-free manner. However, if end-to-end anastomosis of the PD is not possible due to tissue loss, a vein graft may be used to bridge this gap. Several reports describe success with forearm vein grafts to span a wide area of duct discontinuity. When possible, this should be considered with placement of an indwelling salivary stent for 4 to 6 weeks. Interposition vein grafting should be performed if the surgical team believes the outcome would be at least equivalent to other treatment options (eg, duct ligation). If this option is offered to the patient, the risks and benefits of a vein graft should be reviewed in comparison to duct ligation.[20–22]
3. *Possible PD ligation or reimplantation*: The patient is informed that when the exploration reveals significant injury to the proximal duct, repair is not possible, and ligation is performed to induce gland atrophy and to prevent a sialocele or fistula. For distal injuries, the risks associated with reimplantation of the duct can include facial nerve injury or duct stenosis.
4. Intraoperative botulinum toxin injection should be discussed with patients. This can be a valuable tool to prevent postoperative sialoceles and salivary fistulas (see later discussion).

Preoperative Discussion: Anesthesia Team

Long-acting paralytics that would prevent facial nerve monitoring must be avoided during wound exploration. In addition, antisialagogues (atropine or glycopyrrolate) should be held if possible because the identification of the proximal stump of the transected PD often depends on expressing saliva with massage of the gland.[17] Perioperative antibiotics that cover gram positives and oral flora should be given at the beginning of the case.

Operating Room Set-Up: Instrumentation

1. Salivary duct dilators: To cannulate the papilla of Stensen duct (**Fig. 5**). Lacrimal probes may also be used.
2. Sialendoscopy setup (see **Fig. 5**): Use of the all-in-one interventional sialendoscopes (range, 0.8 mm to 1.6 mm) to ensure proper identification of the distal end of the duct and avoid a false passage or sidewall perforation of the duct.[6,23–25]
3. Irrigation setup: An angiocath connected to a syringe is used to irrigate and identify the distal end of the duct—saline is preferred over methylene blue, which can stain the surrounding tissues. An IV extension tubing should also be included along with a 10-cc syringe and saline for irrigation during sialendoscopy to allow visualization of the duct and identification of the cut ends of the duct on exploration.
4. Catheters are placed to span the defect and prevent back-wall placement of sutures during microsurgical repair of the PD. Commercially available stents are available but other commonly available materials may also be used[24] (**Table 1**). (Video 1) https://ndorsellc174.sharefile.com/share/view/sc887bd2e723943edb076282586a26165
5. Microvascular instruments for duct and nerve repair (if applicable).

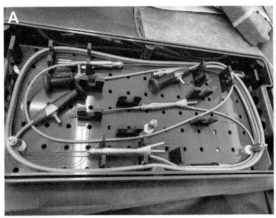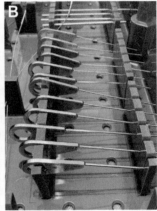

Fig. 5. Sialendoscopic Instrumentation. 5A-Sialendoscope 5B-Salivary duct dilators. Sialoendoscopic instruments can be used in the diagnosis and repair of acute or subacute PD injuries.

6. Oral tray with oral retractors and mouth props to visualize Stensen duct for cannulation.
7. Continuous nerve monitor system: Branches of the upper and lower divisions of the facial nerve are monitored to prevent injury and to identify branches for repair.
8. Operating microscope or loupe magnification (2.5×–3.5×, recommended)

Technique for Repair by Zone of Injury

A. Parenchymal/Zone A Injury: The wound exploration in all cases must involve cannulation of the PD and determination of integrity, followed by irrigation and wound debridement. The fascia of the PG must be meticulously repaired with absorbable suture material, followed by layered closure of the superficial musculoaponeurotic system and skin.[26] The duct may be stented for 1 to 2 weeks to maintain patency and prevent duct obstruction given the resulting edema during the initial healing period.[11,15,18,27]

Table 1
Stents for use in parotid duct injury

Instrument Name	Diameter (mm)
Radiopaque Pebax Walvekar Salivary Duct Stent (WSS) with Guidewire (1.4mm WSS with Irrigating Catheter)	0.6, 1.0, 1.2, and 1.4 mm
Polyurethane leadercath central venous catheter[29]	1.5
Double J stent urethral catheter[50]	2
Size 6 feeding tube[28]	2
Spring-Wire Guide from an arterial line kit[51]	0.64
Epidural catheter[30,31]	1.6
Intracatheter[21]	1.33
Small angiocatheter[17]	20–22 gauge
F4 Fogarty Embolectomy Catheter with a Microvascular Clamp[52]	1.333

B. Zone B Injury (**Fig. 6**): The distal duct is usually identified first via intraoral cannulation. Sialendoscopy can assist when there is resistance to passage of probes to avoid creation of a false passage rather than the identification of the true distal end. The proximal end should be in the same plane as the distal end unless there is a large defect or significant maceration/injury of the soft tissues (see **Fig. 4**; **Fig. 6**). The proximal and distal ends must be dissected free of surrounding soft tissues to achieve a tension free closure (**Fig. 3**). A stent is passed through distal end into the wound, bridging the defect and advanced to proximal stump. Several types of stents can be used appropriate to the diameter of the duct (see **Table 1**).[15,27–32] The duct is repaired over the stent under microscope or loupe magnification. Nylon suture (7–0 to 10–0) is the often-reported material of choice in case series.[18,26,27,33] The stent is kept long enough to exit the papilla of Stensen duct so that it can be secured to the buccal mucosa. Recommended duration of stenting is 2 to 6 weeks.[12,26,27,32,34] If tension-free repair of the PD cannot be achieved, or both ends cannot be identified, the proximal duct must be ligated to allow for gland atrophy.[11] A wide gap between the duct ends can also be spanned with a vein interposition graft.[20–22] Repair of the parotid fascia and more superficial soft tissues proceeds as described for Zone A reconstruction. A parotidectomy is not unreasonable to consider if duct repair is not possible due to inability to identify the proximal cut end of the duct. The feasibility of a parotidectomy and timing will depend on the type of injury. For traumatic injuries, it may be prudent to wait due to open contamination of the buccal space.

C. Zone C (or Distal Zone B) Injury involves the distal end of the PD. The viable distal end of the PD must be reimplanted into the oral cavity. It is diverted and passed through the buccinator muscle, and a new papilla is widely marsupialized, and stented to maintain patency.[26,27]

Additional wound care may also involve passive or suction bulb drain placement. Intraoperative botulinum toxin A injections into the gland parenchyma have been applied in situations where the risk of fistula or sialocele development is deemed

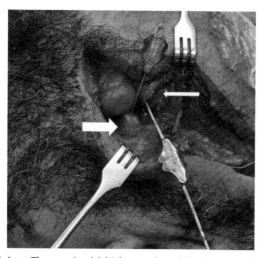

Fig. 6. Zone B PD injury. The proximal (*thick arrow*) and distal ends (*thin arrow*) are cannulated with lacrimal probes. They are found in the same plane and will be dissected free of soft tissue for tension-free approximation and repair.

high.[23] By blocking cholinergic activity, healing of the gland is promoted. Other means to decrease salivation postoperatively include the use of oral antisialogogues, prolonged pressure dressing application, or a period without oral intake; however, these approaches come with systemic side effects that can be difficult for patients to tolerate.[3,24] A pressure dressing applied for 24 to 48 hours postoperatively is a reasonable consideration.

Sialodendoscopy and Parotid Duct Injuries

Sialendoscopy, with its ability to evaluate and treat ductal pathology, has brought to the clinical spectrum the possibility of managing many complex salivary gland conditions such as ductal stenosis and strictures related to inflammatory and autoimmune salivary gland disease, such as radioactive iodine-induced sialadenitis, Sjogren's sialadenitis, and juvenile recurrent parotitis.[35] Sialendoscopy as relates to the management of PD injuries can be an adjunctive tool. However, interventional sialendoscopy can be the cause of PD trauma as well, especially in the setting of friable tissues that are encountered in acute or delayed trauma scenarios.[35,36] Minor ductal trauma can occur because of inadvertent ductal rupture or injury because of traumatic dilation. In this scenario, the ductal injury can be clearly visualized endoscopically. These ductal injuries will resolve without intervention. When possible, a guidewire can be placed beyond the site of injury under endoscopic visualization followed by a stent fashioned to length.

Late Management

Parotid fistula and sialocele are late complications of unrecognized or inappropriately managed PG and PD injuries.[6,23–25] Late complications may also occur when the repair of PD injury is not successful. Parotid fistula is a tract that communicates between salivary tissue and skin and results in the external drainage of saliva. It usually develops within the first week after injury.[15] Sialocele is a fluid-filled cavity that results from saliva extravasation. In contrast to parotid fistula, sialoceles develop more slowly, usually presenting 8 to 14 days after the initial trauma.[2] Sialoceles present a soft and nontender mass in the mandibular ramus region. Sialocele can convert into a fistula if it ruptures through the skin. In addition to a physical examination, a fluid aspirate analysis can be ordered. Amylase levels above 10,000 U/L is diagnostic of sialocele or salivary fistula.[26] Ultrasonography is often the first-line imaging modality used in evaluation.[23,34,37] MRI sialography can also provide valuable information; in this type of imaging, saliva is reconstructed to delineate the ductal anatomy. It is noninvasive and can provide valuable information to plan further management, that is, surgical exploration, conservative treatment, or gland excision. Sialendoscopy can readily assess duct patency after PD repair. Endoscopic view of the suture line after duct repair (shown in video clip 2) demonstrates good patency post repair (Video 2).

Conservative management is favored as the initial treatment of both fistulas and sialoceles. The main principles of medical management are a combination of antibiotics to decrease bacterial overgrowth, pressure dressing application, repeat aspirations in the case of sialoceles, and antisialagogues.[3,15,17] Antibiotics should cover *Staphylococcus aureus*, *Haemophilus influenzae*, and anaerobes.[38] The major innervation to the PG is via cholinergic parasympathetic secretomotor fibers. Anticholinergic medications, such as propantheline, have been successfully used to decrease salivary secretions during the healing period.[15] Unfortunately, these medications are associated with unpleasant side effects, such as xerostomia, urinary retention, tachycardia, and fatigue, thus, limiting their use. In addition, low-dose radiation has been used to induce fibrosis and decrease salivary flow.[39] This modality has been abandoned due to its adverse effects and potential for carcinogenesis.

An attractive alternative is Botulinum toxin, produced by *Clostridium botulinum*,[40–42] which causes selective chemical denervation by inhibiting the release of the acetylcholine at the junction of cholinergic autonomics controlling salivary flow. Suppression of salivary flow begins 1 to 2 weeks after injection and can last from 3 to 6 months or longer, which allows more than adequate healing time.[43] Both prospective and retrospective studies have shown an adequate response to nonsurgical, conservative management.[2,4] Botulinum toxin A injection has risen higher in importance as an initial conservative management choice given a low side effect profile and ease of administration. Ultrasound guidance can be used both to direct sialocele aspiration and specifically target intraglandular injection[25,37,43] but has not been utilized in all reports.[6,23,24,44]

If conservative medical management of late complications of parotid trauma fails, surgical strategies aimed at suppressing or diverting parotid secretions must be considered.[15] Tympanic neurectomy entails autonomic parasympathetic denervation via transection of Jacobsen nerve, a branch of cranial nerve IX, aimed at diminishing PG secretion.[45] This suppressive effect is temporary, usually lasting several weeks to months.[15] Direct surgical management of failed conservative measures of sialocele or fistula includes reexploration of the wound and depending on findings, reconstruction of an unrepaired ductal injury, duct ligation or reimplantation as outlined in the acute setting.[2,46] Sialendoscopy can be used as a diagnostic modality to confirm ductal injury intraoperatively, with endoscopic findings guiding further decision-making during wound exploration.[34] Sialendoscopy also offers the possibility of decreasing the extent of dissection needed to identify the duct ends, thereby minimizing the risk to nearby structures.[34,47–49] Intraoperative (or in the immediate postoperative period) botulinum toxin A has been cited as a means to decrease postoperative fistula or sialocele formation in these cases.[23]

Ultimately, if medical management and conservative reexploration fail, parotidectomy should be considered while keeping in mind a higher risk of complications due to fibrosis and scarring from chronic inflammation.

SUMMARY

Diagnosis and treatment of PG and duct injuries require a significant commitment of clinical resources. Given the rarity of this injury compared with other types of facial trauma, familiarity with key diagnostic steps and classification schemes that inform decision-making is important for all surgeons who may be called to evaluate patients with penetrating cheek trauma. The addition of endoscopic tools used in more elective settings has been an important adjunct in acute and delayed parotid trauma presentations adding to the safety and improved outcomes for patients.

CLINICS CARE POINTS

- Bedside diagnosis of a transected PD can be accomplished with proper instrumentation but the optimal setting for injury identification is the operating room.
- Consent for cheek wound exploration should be comprehensive, anticipating all possible duct injury patterns.

- Botulinum toxin injection, with or without ultrasound guidance, can decrease the length of duration of salivary fistula or sialoceles that may complicate treatment.

DISCLOSURE

Dr R.R. Walvekar–Hood Laboratories, Pembroke MA–Walvekar Salivary Stent (Consultant/Inventor).

SUPPLEMENTARY DATA

Supplementary data related to this article can be found online at https://doi.org/10.1016/j.otc.2023.05.007.

REFERENCES

1. Lewis G, Knottenbelt JD. Parotid duct injury: is immediate surgical repair necessary? Injury 1991;22(5):407–9.
2. Parekh D, Glezerson G, Stewart M, et al. Post-traumatic parotid fistulae and sialoceles. A prospective study of conservative management in 51 cases. Ann Surg 1989;209(1):105–11.
3. Lazaridou M, Iliopoulos C, Antoniades K, et al. Salivary gland trauma: a review of diagnosis and treatment. Craniomaxillofac Trauma Reconstr 2012;5(4):189–96.
4. Tachmes L, Woloszyn T, Marini C, et al. Parotid gland and facial nerve trauma: a retrospective review. J Trauma 1990;30(11):1395–8.
5. Landau R, Stewart M. Conservative management of post-traumatic parotid fistulae and sialoceles: a prospective study. Br J Surg 1985;72(1):42–4.
6. Costan VV, Dabija MG, Ciofu ML, et al. A Functional Approach to Posttraumatic Salivary Fistula Treatment: The Use of Botulinum Toxin. J Craniofac Surg 2019;30(3):871–5.
7. Tsai CH, Ting CC, Wu SY, et al. Clinical significance of buccal branches of the facial nerve and their relationship with the emergence of Stensen's duct: An anatomical study on adult Taiwanese cadavers. J Cranio-Maxillo-Fac Surg 2019;47(11):1809–18.
8. Stringer MD, Mirjalili SA, Meredith SJ, et al. Redefining the surface anatomy of the parotid duct: an in vivo ultrasound study. Plast Reconstr Surg 2012;130(5):1032–7.
9. Goncalves M, Mantsopoulos K, Schapher M, et al. Ultrasound in the diagnosis of parotid duct obstruction not caused by sialolithiasis: diagnostic value in reference to direct visualization with sialendoscopy. Dentomaxillofac Radiol 2021;50(3):20200261.
10. Zenk J, Hosemann WG, Iro H. Diameters of the main excretory ducts of the adult human submandibular and parotid gland: a histologic study. Oral Surg Oral Med Oral Pathol Oral Radiol Endod 1998;85(5):576–80.
11. Van Sickels JE. Management of parotid gland and duct injuries. Oral Maxillofac Surg Clin North Am 2009;21(2):243–6.
12. Van Sickels JE. Parotid duct injuries. Oral Surg Oral Med Oral Pathol 1981;52(4):364–7.
13. Perry M, Morris C. Advanced trauma life support (ATLS) and facial trauma: can one size fit all? Part 2: ATLS, maxillofacial injuries and airway management dilemmas. Int J Oral Maxillofac Surg 2008;37(4):309–20.

14. Cho DY, Willborg BE, Lu GN. Management of Traumatic Soft Tissue Injuries of the Face. Semin Plast Surg 2021;35(4):229–37.
15. Gordin EA, Daniero JJ, Krein H, et al. Parotid gland trauma. Facial Plast Surg 2010;26(6):504–10.
16. Tisch M, Maier S, Maier H. Penetrating Trauma to the Parotid Gland. Facial Plast Surg 2015;31(4):376–81.
17. Steinberg MJ, Herrera AF. Management of parotid duct injuries. Oral Surg Oral Med Oral Pathol Oral Radiol Endod 2005;99(2):136–41.
18. Lewkowicz AA, Hasson O, Nahlieli O. Traumatic injuries to the parotid gland and duct. J Oral Maxillofac Surg 2002;60(6):676–80.
19. Greywoode JD, Ho HH, Artz GJ, et al. Management of traumatic facial nerve injuries. Facial Plast Surg 2010;26(6):511–8.
20. Heymans O, Nelissen X, Medot M, et al. Microsurgical repair of Stensen's duct using an interposition vein graft. J Reconstr Microsurg 1999;15(2):105–7, discussion 107-108.
21. Awana M, Arora SS, Arora S, et al. Reconstruction of a traumatically transected Stensen's duct using facial vein graft. Ann Maxillofac Surg 2015;5(1):96–9.
22. Liang CC, Jeng SF, Yeh MC, et al. Reconstruction of traumatic Stensen duct defect using a vein graft as a conduit: two case reports. Ann Plast Surg 2004;52(1):102–4.
23. Kopec T, Wierzbicka M, Szyfter W. Stensen's duct injuries: the role of sialendoscopy and adjuvant botulinum toxin injection. Wideochir Inne Tech Maloinwazyjne 2013;8(2):112–6.
24. Arnaud S, Batifol D, Goudot P, et al. Nonsurgical management of traumatic injuries of the parotid gland and duct using type a botulinum toxin. Plast Reconstr Surg 2006;117(7):2426–30.
25. Gok G, Michl P, Williams MD, et al. Ultrasound-guided botulinum toxin injection to treat a parotid fistula following gunshot injury. J R Army Med Corps 2015;161(1):64–6.
26. Shupak RP, Williams FC, Kim RY. Management of Salivary Gland Injury. Oral Maxillofac Surg Clin North Am 2021;33(3):343–50.
27. McElwee TJ, Poche JN, Sowder JC, et al. Management of Acute Facial Nerve and Parotid Injuries. Facial Plast Surg 2021;37(4):490–9.
28. Mardani M, Arabion H. Surgical Management of Parotid Duct Injury Using a Feeding Tube. Ann Maxillofac Surg 2020;10(2):472–4.
29. Hills AJ, Kannan RY, Williams M. Seldinger technique in repair of the parotid duct. Br J Oral Maxillofac Surg 2019;57(1):85–7.
30. Kumar SR, Hiremath V, Patil AG, et al. Surgical management of Stenson's duct injury using epidural catheter: a novel technique. Niger J Clin Pract 2013;16(2):266–8.
31. Sujeeth S, Dindawar S. Parotid duct repair using an epidural catheter. Int J Oral Maxillofac Surg 2011;40(7):747–8.
32. Ozturk MB, Barutca SA, Keskin ES, et al. Parotid Duct Repair with Intubation Tube: Technical Note. Ann Maxillofac Surg 2017;7(1):129–31.
33. Hallock GG. Microsurgical repair of the parotid duct. Microsurgery 1992;13(5):243–6.
34. Koch M, Iro H, Bozzato A, et al. Sialendoscopy-assisted microsurgical repair of traumatic transection of Stensen's duct. Laryngoscope 2013;123(12):3074–7.
35. Jackson EM, Walvekar RR. Surgical Techniques for the Management of Parotid Salivary Duct Strictures. Atlas Oral Maxillofac Surg Clin North Am 2018;26(2):93–8.

36. Chandra SR. Sialoendoscopy: Review and Nuances of Technique. J Maxillofac Oral Surg 2019;18(1):1–10.

37. Tighe D, Williams M, Howett D. Treatment of iatrogenic sialoceles and fistulas in the parotid gland with ultrasound-guided injection of botulinum toxin A. Br J Oral Maxillofac Surg 2015;53(1):97–8.

38. Brook I. The bacteriology of salivary gland infections. Oral Maxillofac Surg Clin North Am 2009;21(3):269–74.

39. Wallenborn WM, Hsu YT, Olinger BR. The experimental production of parotid gland atrophy. Laryngoscope 1968;78(8):1314–28.

40. Marchese Ragona R, Blotta P, Pastore A, et al. Management of parotid sialocele with botulinum toxin. Laryngoscope 1999;109(8):1344–6.

41. Marchese-Ragona R, Marioni G, Restivo DA, et al. The role of botulinum toxin in postparotidectomy fistula treatment. A technical note. Am J Otolaryngol 2006; 27(3):221–4.

42. Vargas H, Galati LT, Parnes SM. A pilot study evaluating the treatment of postparotidectomy sialoceles with botulinum toxin type A. Arch Otolaryngol Head Neck Surg 2000;126(3):421–4.

43. Ellies M, Gottstein U, Rohrbach-Volland S, et al. Reduction of salivary flow with botulinum toxin: extended report on 33 patients with drooling, salivary fistulas, and sialadenitis. Laryngoscope 2004;114(10):1856–60.

44. von Lindern JJ, Niederhagen B, Appel T, et al. New prospects in the treatment of traumatic and postoperative parotid fistulas with type A botulinum toxin. Plast Reconstr Surg 2002;109(7):2443–5.

45. Davis WE, Holt GR, Templer JW. Parotid fistula and tympanic neurectomy. Am J Surg 1977;133(5):587–9.

46. Hu CY, Shang ZJ, Qin X, et al. Application of Delayed Surgical Managements in Patients with Stensen's Duct Injury. Curr Med Sci 2018;38(3):519–23.

47. Wu CB, Xi H, Zhang LM, et al. Sialendoscopy-assisted treatment of trauma to Stensen's duct: technical note. Br J Oral Maxillofac Surg 2015;53(1):102–3.

48. Wu CB, Sun HJ, Li FL, et al. Sialendoscopy-Assisted Treatment of Stensen's Duct Injury: A Case Series. J Oral Maxillofac Surg 2020;78(9):1595.

49. Man CB, Patel R, Karavidas K. Intraoperative sialendoscopy to assist with and confirm repair of Stensen's duct. Br J Oral Maxillofac Surg 2017;55(7):e45–6.

50. Aloosi SN, Khoshnaw N, Ali SM, et al. Surgical management of Stenson's duct injury by using double J stent urethral catheter. Int J Surg Case Rep 2015; 17:75–8.

51. Demian N, Curtis W. A simple technique for cannulation of the parotid duct. J Oral Maxillofac Surg 2008;66(7):1532–3.

52. Etoz A, Tuncel U, Ozcan M. Parotid duct repair by use of an embolectomy catheter with a microvascular clamp. Plast Reconstr Surg 2006;117(1):330–1.

Laryngeal Trauma

Claude Nganzeu, MD[a,b], Antoinette Esce, MD[a,b],
Sara Abu-Ghanem, MD, MmedSc[c], Duncan A. Meiklejohn, MD[a,b],
H. Steven Sims, MD, FACS[d,*]

KEYWORDS

- Laryngeal trauma • Airway • Fracture • Thyroid • Cricoid

KEY POINTS

- Traumatic laryngeal injuries are rare but potentially lethal injuries.
- Management of laryngeal trauma is based on severity and multiple classification systems exist.
- Early intervention to preserve airway and laryngeal function improves long-term outcomes.

INTRODUCTION

The larynx is a complex structure consisting of multiple interlocking cartilages and a single sesamoid bone and is necessary for a functional voice, airway, and swallow. Fractures of the laryngotracheal complex are rare, with incidence between 1 in 5000 and 1 in 137,000 Emergency Department (ED) visits.[1–5] Airway management is critical and requires careful consideration of all clinical factors on an individualized basis.

HISTORY AND DEFINITIONS
Classification Systems of Laryngeal Injuries

Several classification systems have been proposed to assist with diagnosing and managing laryngeal injury. The mechanism is usually classified as blunt or penetrating, with blunt force being most common.[5–8] Lynch and colleagues were the first to describe a laryngeal cartilage fracture classification system based on injury location in 1951; this was modified by Nahum in 1969.[8] In 1980, Schaefer described a

[a] Division of Otolaryngology–Head and Neck Surgery, Department of Surgery, University of New Mexico; [b] Department of Surgery ENT 1, University of New Mexico, MSC10, 5610, Albuquerque, NM 87131, USA; [c] Laryngology and Bronchoesophagology, Department of Otolaryngology, SUNY Downstate & Maimonides Health, 185 Montague Street, 5th Floor, Brooklyn, NY 11220, USA; [d] University of Illinois Hospital and Health Service Systems, 1855 West Taylor Street, Room 3.87, Chicago, IL 60612, USA
* Corresponding author.
E-mail address: hssims@uic.edu

Otolaryngol Clin N Am 56 (2023) 1039–1053
https://doi.org/10.1016/j.otc.2023.06.001
0030-6665/23/© 2023 Elsevier Inc. All rights reserved.

classification system based on the severity of injury.[9] Patients were evaluated using a combination of indirect laryngoscopy (mirror examination) and neck tissue x-ray, with later cases including computed tomography (CT) to further characterize the extent of injury. Those with an unstable airway were examined via direct laryngoscopy following tracheotomy.[9] Fuhrman later modified this classification to include laryngotracheal separation (**Table 1**).[6] Verschueren and colleagues[5] modified the Schaefer-Fuhrman classification in 2006 to include the use of CT imaging (**Table 2**).

CRITICAL ANATOMIC DEFINITIONS

The laryngotracheal complex is located in the anterior midline neck and is shielded from external trauma by the mandible, sternum, and the spine.[10]

The larynx extends from the base of the tongue to the trachea, roughly between the C3 and C6 vertebrae in adult men and slightly higher in women.[10] The laryngeal skeleton is composed of multiple cartilages and the hyoid bone, which are suspended from the mandible and skull base by ligamentous attachments (**Figs. 1–3**).[10–12] There are 3 large unpaired laryngeal cartilages; the epiglottis, the thyroid cartilage, and cricoid cartilage, as well as smaller, paired cartilages; the arytenoid, corniculate, and cuneiform cartilages.

The thyroid cartilage consists of 2 roughly quadrangular laminae of hyaline cartilage that fuse anteriorly, with a wider angle in women (see **Figs. 1–3**).[11–14] Intrinsic laryngeal muscles are located within and around the thyroid cartilage. The intrinsic laryngeal muscles function to adduct, abduct, and change the shape and tension of the vocal folds.[10,13–15] Thyroid cartilage fractures can cause changes in the shape, position, and mobility of the vocal folds leading to dysphonia and/or airway compromise.[7,8]

The cricoid cartilage is connected to the trachea and thyroid cartilage by membranous attachments (see **Figs. 1–3**).[10–15] Cricoid fractures may cause significant swelling or hematoma at or below the level of the vocal folds.

The arytenoid cartilages are paired cartilages positioned atop the cricoid lamina. Arytenoid movement by the intrinsic laryngeal muscles is predominantly responsible for mobility of the vocal folds.[10,13,15] Dislocation of the arytenoids can cause foreshortening of the vocal folds and affect phonation, or paralysis of the vocal folds and limitation of phonation and/or airway.[8]

The epiglottis is a leaf-shaped elastic cartilage located within the larynx at its anterior and superior aspect (see **Fig. 3**).[10,12–15] Injury to the superior larynx can cause epiglottic hematoma leading to stridor, dysphonia, respiratory distress, and airway compromise.[8]

Table 1	
Fuhrman-Schaefer classification of laryngeal injuries, with permission[8]	
Stage	**Injury**
I	Minor laryngeal hematoma, edema, laceration; no detectable fracture
II	Edema, hematoma, mucosal disruption with no exposed cartilage, nondisplaced fractures
III	Significant edema, noted mucosal disruption, exposed cartilage with or without cord immobility, displaced fractures
IV	Significant edema, noted mucosal disruption, exposed cartilage with or without cord immobility, displaced fractures with 2 or more fracture lines, skeletal instability/anterior commissure trauma
V	Complete laryngotracheal separation

Table 2 Legacy Emanuel Medical Center laryngeal injury classification, with permission[8]	
Stage	**Diagnostic Findings**
I	Minor airway Symptoms ± voice changes No fractures Small lacerations
II	Airway compromise Nondisplaced fractures No cartilage exposure Voice changes ± Subcutaneous emphysema
III	Airway compromise Edema Mucosal lacerations Palpable laryngeal fractures Exposed cartilage Subcutaneous emphysemas Voice changes
IV	Airway compromise Mucosal lacerations Exposed cartilage Palpable displaced laryngeal fractures with skeletal instability Subcutaneous emphysemas Voice changes

The larynx is innervated bilaterally by the superior and recurrent laryngeal branches of the vagus nerve (cranial nerve X).[10,16] The superior laryngeal nerve is divided into external and internal branches. The external branch of the superior laryngeal nerve (EBSLN) follows the course of the superior thyroid vessels and provides motor innervation to the cricothyroid muscle, which acts to lengthen and shorten the vocal folds. The internal branch of the superior laryngeal nerve (IBSLN) penetrates the thyrohyoid membrane and provides sensory innervation to the internal laryngeal structures superior to the vocal folds.[16] Injury to the EBSLN disrupts maximal lengthening and tension of the vocal folds, limiting the ability to produce higher pitched voice. Injury to the IBSLN causes sensory deficits in the supraglottic laryngeal mucosa, which may result in aspiration and dysphagia.[16]

The recurrent laryngeal nerve (RLN) provides motor innervation to all the intrinsic laryngeal muscles except the cricothyroid muscle, and provides sensory innervation to structures inferior to the vocal folds and infraglottic surface of the vocal folds. The right RLN branches from the vagus nerve at the level of the T1 to T2 vertebrae and loops under the right subclavian artery, traveling posterosuperiorly in the tracheoesophageal groove.[16] The left RLN branches from the vagus nerve at the aortic arch, loops posteriorly around the arch and travels superiorly in the tracheoesophageal groove.[17] On both sides, the nerve enters the larynx posterior to the cricothyroid joint, where the inferior thyroid cornu articulates with the cricoid cartilage. It is particularly susceptible to traumatic injury at this location.[18]

CLINICAL EVALUATION AND MANAGEMENT
History and Physical

Providers should have a high index of suspicion for laryngeal injury when patients present with trauma to the anterior neck. Blunt force trauma from sports or motor vehicle

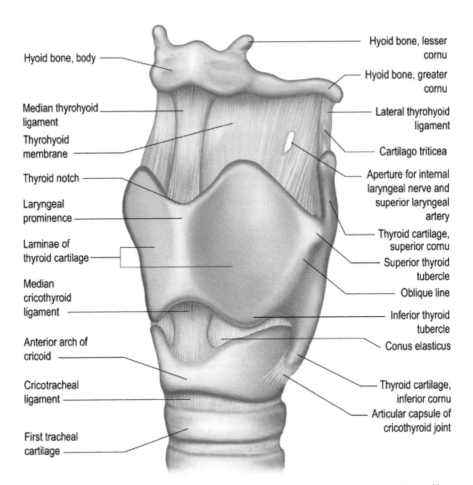

Fig. 1. Anterolateral view of the laryngeal cartilages and ligaments, with permission.[11]

accidents is the most common mechanism of injury to the laryngeal cartilage, although the incidence of vehicular etiology has markedly decreased due to improvements in car safety features.[19] Other mechanisms of injury to the larynx include falls, hanging or strangulation attempts, "clothesline" injuries, and penetrating injury (**Fig. 4**).[20] Hoarseness, respiratory distress, dysphagia, crepitus, hemoptysis, anterior neck pain, and subcutaneous emphysema or crepitus in the neck should heighten suspicion for laryngeal injury. However, it is important to note that some patients with mild laryngeal injuries can be asymptomatic.[21] Patients with external laryngeal trauma often present with associated injuries in the head, neck, or chest. Plain films, CT, or CT angiography of the head, neck, or chest may be indicated to rule out pulmonary or vascular injuries.[22]

For patients with a clinically stable airway, flexible bedside laryngoscopy should be used to visualize the mucosal surface of the larynx,[19,23] although this should never delay more emergent interventions. Flexible laryngoscopy may identify edema, hematoma, lacerations, and exposed cartilage and can also assess vocal fold mobility and airway patency. Esophagoscopy and fluoroscopic imaging can be used to identify esophageal injuries, which are encountered in only 4% to 6% of laryngeal fractures but may cause significant morbidity or even mortality.[19,24]

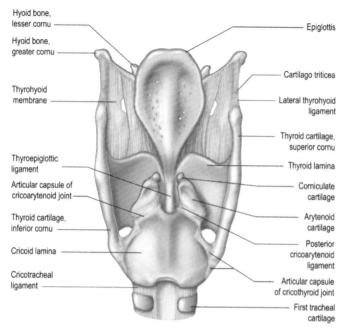

Fig. 2. Posterior view of the laryngeal cartilages and ligaments, with permission.[11]

Either patients with incidentally found laryngotracheal injury on CT imaging or patients with voice or respiratory symptoms following trauma to the neck should undergo a complete physical examination including careful palpation of the laryngeal framework and bedside flexible laryngoscopy. Laryngeal injuries may evolve over hours, especially those caused by blunt force, and identifying mucosal injuries before airway compromise is crucial.[7]

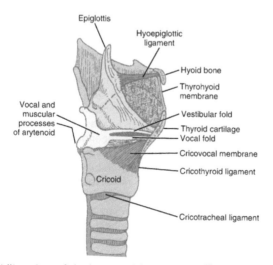

Fig. 3. Sagittal midline view of the larynx, with permission.[12]

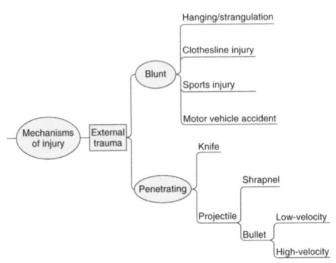

Fig. 4. Mechanisms of laryngeal cartilage injury, with permission.[20]

IMAGING

There is no clear consensus regarding the use of CT imaging in the diagnosis of laryngeal cartilage fractures.[19,23,25] Much of the literature on laryngeal fractures is based on a detailed 27-year case series from Schaefer and colleagues published in the 1990s,[4] in which CT scans were only routinely used during the last 10 years of the series.

The sensitivity of CT imaging is limited by the various patterns of laryngeal cartilage ossification in patients.[26] In fact, 2-dimensional axial images can miss upward of 12% of laryngeal cartilage fractures and nearly half of hyoid bone fractures.[27] These rates are improved with additional multidimensional renderings. In patients with minimal symptoms, stable clinical examinations, and an evaluation consistent with Schaefer Stage I or II injury, dedicated CT imaging for laryngeal fractures may not be necessary. Newer classification frameworks such as the Legacy Emanuel Medical Center laryngeal injury classification incorporate the degree of fracture displacement into their injury levels (see **Table 2**).[5]

AIRWAY MANAGEMENT

Laryngeal cartilage fractures can be fatal if not managed appropriately.[23,25] The opinions regarding airway management in patients with intermediate severity laryngeal fractures are evolving. However, establishing and maintaining a secure airway in a safe and atraumatic manner is the first step in managing any of these complex injuries.[23] Patients who do not show signs of impending airway compromise do not require immediate invasive airway control; however, they should be observed over several hours in an intensive care setting with focused serial examinations including flexible laryngoscopy. Patients with severe blunt trauma, displaced fractures, and/or extensive mucosal lacerations or injury are at particular risk of decompensating.[7]

Either patients in respiratory distress secondary to laryngotracheal trauma or those with polytrauma and concomitant laryngotracheal injury requiring immediate airway control for other reasons, pose a clinical challenge. This stems from difficulties visualizing the airway due to edema, hematoma, or distortion of the normal anatomy.[23,25] Intubation by an inexperienced physician can result in significant consequences such as creation of a false passage, further soft tissue damage, disruption of anatomy, or potentially life-threatening airway compromise.[7,21,23] Emergent intubation must be performed by an experienced physician under direct visualization; additionally, the airway should be intact with minimal visible injury.[7,23] Interestingly, often times, patients present to the ED already intubated. After the innovations of Dr Peter Safar and the Freedom House Paramedics from Pittsburgh, most specifically the creation of the first paramedics in the United States (**Fig. 5**), first responders may secure the airway in the field, including intubation.[28]

If intubation is unsuccessful or the airway is deemed unstable, a surgical airway is indicated.[19] Patients with significant mucosal injury or severely displaced fractures should undergo awake tracheostomy. Traditional emergent cricothyrotomy or endotracheal intubation carry the risk of separating the trachea from the cricoid cartilage with attempted passage of an endotracheal tube from above the cricoid, a potentially lethal event, which can occur in cases of occult traumatic laryngotracheal separation.[3,4,6] Select patients with a stable airway who require surgical intervention may be safely intubated in the operating room and then converted to a tracheostomy as necessary. Interestingly, the existing data show that most patients do not require any invasive airway management, immediate or otherwise. For example, in a 15-year retrospective case series of 56 patients by Wang and colleagues,[25] 35 patients did not require any invasive airway control. Generally, the role for supralaryngeal airway devices is extremely limited.

TREATMENT

The main goals in the management of laryngeal cartilage fractures are to restore the laryngeal skeletal framework, preserve high-quality phonation, and protect respiratory function.[7,23,24] The best results are achieved by the early recognition of the laryngeal injury, rapid establishment of a safe airway if necessary, and managing promptly based on the extent of the injury.[7,23,25] Patients who were treated within 48 hours had better voice and airway outcomes compared with patients who underwent delayed intervention.[3,23,29]

CONSERVATIVE MANAGEMENT

For patients with reversible injuries such as mild edema, small hematoma, or minor lacerations (Stage I injuries), Schaefer proposes a conservative management algorithm

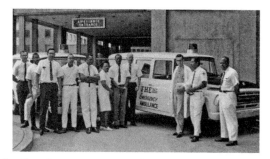

Fig. 5. Some of the first Emergency Responders were part of the Freedom House jobs training program in Pittsburgh's African-American Hill District. (Source: Caligiuri and Curto family papers and photographs, 2019.0215, Thomas and Katherine Detre Library and Archives, Senator John Heinz History Center. Gift of Virginia 'Ginny' Caligiuri.)

with a 12 to 24-hour airway watch period. Interventions in this period include head of bed elevation, voice rest, and steroid therapy to decrease laryngeal edema, as well as inhaled cool mist or humidified air to decrease ciliary paralysis and improve the management of secretions.[7,24] Acid reducing agents such as histamine blockers and proton pump inhibitors have been proposed but there is no definitive evidence for or against managing reflux.[7] Intuitively, control of irritation from acid and digestive enzymes is likely to show a favorable cost–benefit analysis. The use of laryngoscopy with videostroboscopy is often used during recovery for detailed assessment of vocal fold mobility. Voice and airway outcomes are excellent with conservative management for patients with Stage I injuries.[7,23] Schaefer advocates surgical fixation for Stage II injuries, even with nondisplaced fractures, arguing that nondisplaced fractures may widen days to weeks after the injury and can affect the function of the larynx. This is especially true if the fracture affects the angulated part of the thyroid cartilage.[7] Alternatively, Moonsamy and colleagues[24] recommend nonoperative management of Stage II injuries. Careful consideration of the location of the nondisplaced fracture may aid clinical decision-making, with a lower threshold for repair in fractures involving the anterior angle of the thyroid cartilage. Patients with Stage III to V injuries often require surgical intervention and are more likely to require immediate airway control for impending obstruction, with awake tracheostomy favored if they cannot be safely intubated.[7,30]

CASE 1

A 52-year-old man presented to ED an hour following assault by strangulation reporting symptoms of dysphonia, dysphagia, and odynophagia but denies breathing complaints. On examination, patient was breathing comfortably with no stridor but with a breathy voice. The neck examination revealed anterior neck erythema with diffuse crepitus. Flexible laryngoscopy found minimal pooling of blood in pyriform sinuses, no active bleeding, nonobstructing edema of arytenoids, and right true vocal fold hypomobility. Computed tomography angiography (CTA) of the neck found no vascular injuries, significant subcutaneous air, and fracture of thyroid cartilage with

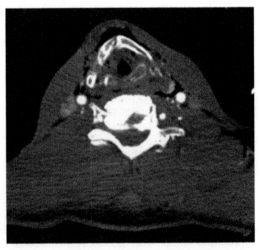

Fig. 6. CT scan of neck axial view, significant subcutaneous air, and minimally displaced fracture of the thyroid cartilage.

minimal displacement (**Fig. 6**). A decision was made to establish a definitive airway and the patient was brought to the operating room (OR) for awake tracheostomy followed by direct laryngoscopy and esophagoscopy and open reduction and internal fixation (ORIF) of the thyroid cartilage fracture (**Fig. 7**). Laryngoscopic findings showed moderate edema and ecchymosis of the supraglottis, no exposed cartilage, and no apparent injuries of the cervical esophagus or subglottis. Patient was admitted for observation and decannulated and discharged 10 days later.

CASE 3

A 39-year-old man presented to the ED with odynophagia following blunt trauma to the anterior neck and strangulation. The patient denied dysphonia, globus sensation, or difficulty breathing. On examination, he was found with tenderness to palpation of the anterior neck at level of the thyroid cartilage with no significant swelling. Flexible laryngoscopy revealed minimal erythema and edema of arytenoid complex with a patent airway and bilateral vocal fold motion. CT scan of the neck found a nondisplaced fracture of the right thyroid cartilage (**Fig. 8**). Patient was admitted to the intensive care unit for overnight airway observation, was kept for eating (nothing by mouth) and was treated with intravenous steroids. Patient was discharged the following day after confirming resolution of laryngeal findings and improved symptoms.

SURGICAL TECHNIQUES

Schaefer in 2013 proposed an algorithm for the management of laryngeal cartilage fractures (**Fig. 9**).[7] In patients for whom surgery is indicated, panendoscopy with direct laryngoscopy, tracheoscopy, and esophagoscopy is recommended to rule out simultaneous injuries of the aerodigestive tract, followed by operative repair of laryngeal injuries.[4,7] For patients with greater than 2 endolaryngeal lacerations or any lacerations involving the free edge of the vocal fold, Schaefer proposes a midline thyrotomy

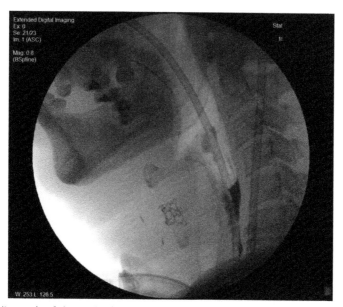

Fig. 7. Radiograph of the neck after ORIF of the cartilage.

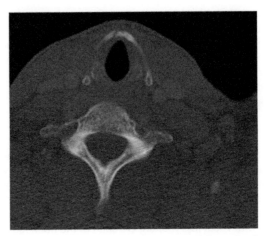

Fig. 8. CT scan of neck axial view, nondisplaced fracture of the right thyroid cartilage.

approach for repair to permit better exposure of the endolarynx (**Fig. 10**).[7] When repairing the endolarynx, it is important to restore the shape of the anterior commissure if distorted or lacerated. This can be achieved by suturing the most anterior portion of the vocal folds and vocal ligament to the outer cartilage perichondrium.[7] To reestablish the laryngeal skeletal framework in laryngeal cartilage fractures, open

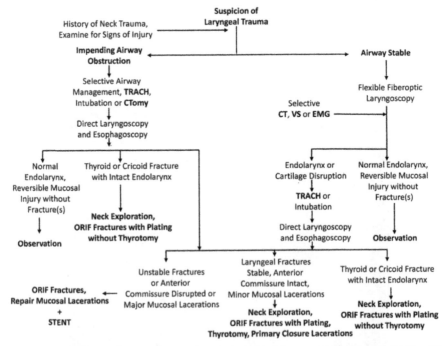

Fig. 9. Algorithm for the treatment of acute laryngeal trauma from Schaefer 2013, with permission.[7] Algorithm for early treatment of acute external laryngeal trauma. CT, computed tomography; CTomy, cricothyrotomy; EMG, electromyography of the larynx; ORIF, open reduction and internal fixation of laryngeal skeletal fractures; STENT, endolaryngeal stent or lumen keeper; TRACH, tracheotomy; VS, videostroboscopy of larynx.

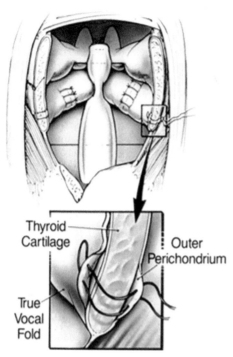

Thyroid Cartilage

Outer Perichondrium

True Vocal Fold

Fig. 10. Primary closure of laryngeal lacerations via a midline thyrotomy. Enlarged image demonstrates the free anterior margin of the true vocal fold sutured to the outer perichondrium of the thyroid cartilage to reestablish tension. (Steven D. Schaefer, The acute surgical treatment of the fractured larynx, Operative Techniques in Otolaryngology-Head and Neck Surgery, 1 (1), 1990, 64-70, https://doi.org/10.1016/S1043-1810(10)80277-5.).

reduction and internal fixation using wires, sutures, miniplates, or mesh is recommended. Macroporous degradable plates, which absorb spontaneously during 1 to 7 years after placement, may be another option for fixation.[31] Severely comminuted fractures or injury to the anterior commissure increase the risk of laryngeal stenosis. In these cases, the lumen of the airway can be kept patent using a lumen keeper or stent.[7,24] However, the use of stents is controversial. Schaefer and colleagues recommend against the use of stents if proper mucosal repair and fracture reduction are achieved as stents can cause infection, granulation tissue formation, scar formation, or pressure necrosis leading airway compromise or poor phonation.[7,24] If stents are used, soft stents rather than hard stents are recommended for the shortest time possible, no more than 2 weeks.[7] Patients with laryngeal stent placement require a tracheostomy for the duration of treatment.

COMPLICATIONS

Complications related to initial injury or subsequent intervention may be classified as acute or chronic.[30] Acute complications include acute airway obstruction, asphyxiation, RLN injury, infection, or postoperative hematoma.[30] Chronic complications include vocal cord paresis/paralysis, dysphonia, laryngeal or tracheal stenosis, or chronic aspiration.[7,30]

LARYNGEAL FRACTURES IN THE PEDIATRIC POPULATION

Laryngeal cartilage fractures are even rarer in the pediatric population. The pediatric larynx is located more superiorly in the neck and is better shielded from direct trauma by the mandible.[32] The laryngeal cartilage in children is more pliable and resistant to fracture.[32,33] The thyroid cartilage does not begin to ossify until around 18 to 20 years old; thus, the pediatric laryngeal cartilage often strains rather than fractures.[27] Although fracture is uncommon, the pediatric population is at higher risk of vocal fold avulsion, glottic edema, and fluid collection from laryngeal cartilage strains.[33]

The most common causes of laryngeal injury in children are furniture injuries, bicycle injuries, and "clothes-line" type trauma.[32,33] Presenting symptoms include hoarseness, dysphagia, hemoptysis, and subcutaneous emphysema. Breathing difficulties and rapid progression of subcutaneous emphysema may signify major injury; however, symptoms of airway distress may be delayed for days after the initial injury. Immediate recognition of the injury and early management of the airway produce better outcomes.[32,34] Airway management is somewhat controversial in the pediatric population but some algorithms do exist, including one from Kurien and colleagues[34] (Fig. 11). The authors favor tracheostomy for major injury and conservative management for minor injuries. Most pediatric patients are eventually decannulated, although they often require multiple interventions.[33]

DISCUSSION
Current Evidence

Current evidence supporting the assessment and management of laryngotracheal trauma comes primarily from case reports and case series. Several articles have attempted to evaluate the problem by looking at large national databases,[1,2] and this is limited by the wide range of presentations and highly varied clinical management. Currently, management relies primarily on an updated version of the nearly

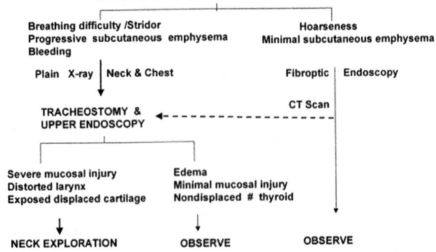

Fig. 11. Algorithm for the treatment of external laryngotracheal trauma in pediatric patients, with permission.[34]

25-year-old Schaefer classification and resulting algorithm (see **Fig. 9**)[7]; however, there remain gaps in the current evidence, including when to perform awake tracheostomy.[5,21,23,25] Currently, the only absolute indication for awake tracheostomy is acute, impending airway compromise. For less severe cases, the method of airway management is still at the discretion of the treating surgeon.

SUMMARY

Traumatic laryngeal fractures are rare but potentially fatal injuries. Successful management lies with early recognition of critical airway signs and symptoms. Radiographic imaging, usually with CT, may identify occult injuries or characterize the extent of laryngeal skeleton injury. Examination of the aerodigestive structures with bedside flexible laryngoscopy is crucial to fully delineate the extent of injury. Establishing a safe airway is the primary goal of acute management of severe laryngeal trauma. This can be done by intubation in the operating room, awake tracheostomy, or if absolutely necessary, careful cricothyroidotomy with conversion to tracheostomy. An experienced provider can perform intubation outside of the operating room if the endolarynx can be visualized and there is no distortion of anatomy. In severe injuries with impending airway obstruction, or if the extent of the injury is unknown, awake tracheostomy is favored due to its greater safety in cases of laryngotracheal separation. Stage I to II injuries can often be managed conservatively but Stage III to V injuries typically require surgical intervention. Patients with extensive endolaryngeal mucosal injury may require laceration repair via midline thyrotomy, and an endolaryngeal stent may provide benefit in select cases. Early intervention results in best phonation, airway, and swallowing outcomes, and most patients requiring tracheostomy are eventually decannulated.

CLINICS CARE POINTS

- Traumatic laryngeal injuries are rare but potentially lethal, and a high index of suspicion is recommended in patients with traumatic injuries to the head and neck.
- The most used classification system is the 1990 Schaefer classification.
- Securing the airway is the essential step in management; traditional airway management techniques may be contraindicated and a laryngeal trauma-specific algorithm should be followed. Awake tracheostomy may be indicated for more severe injuries.
- Early intervention (within 24–48 hours after trauma) is important to optimize long-term outcomes such as voice, speech, swallowing, and airway.

DISCLOSURE

No authors have any relevant commercial or financial conflicts of interest related to this study.

REFERENCES

1. Sethi RKV, Kozin ED, Fagenholz PJ, et al. Epidemiological survey of head and neck injuries and trauma in the United States. Otolaryngol Head Neck Surg 2014;151(5):776–84.
2. Jewett BS, Shockley WW, Rutledge R. External laryngeal trauma analysis of 392 patients. Arch Otolaryngol Head Neck Surg 1999;125(8):877–80.

3. Bent JP, Silver JR, Porubsky ES. Acute laryngeal trauma: a review of 77 patients. Otolaryngol Head Neck Surg 1993;109(3 Pt 1):441–9.
4. Schaefer SD. The acute management of external laryngeal trauma. A 27-year experience. Arch Otolaryngol Head Neck Surg 1992;118(6):598–604.
5. Verschueren DS, Bell RB, Bagheri SC, et al. Management of laryngo-tracheal injuries associated with craniomaxillofacial trauma. J Oral Maxillofac Surg 2006; 64(2):203–14.
6. Fuhrman GM, Stieg FH, Buerk CA. Blunt laryngeal trauma: classification and management protocol. J Trauma 1990;30(1):87–92.
7. Schaefer SD. Management of acute blunt and penetrating external laryngeal trauma. Laryngoscope 2014;124(1):233–44.
8. Elias N, Thomas J, Cheng A. Management of laryngeal trauma. Oral Maxillofacial Surg Clin N Am 2021;33(3):417–27.
9. Schaefer SD. Primary management of laryngeal trauma. Ann Otol Rhinol Laryngol 1982;91(4 Pt 1):399–402.
10. Janfaza P, Joseph B, Nadol JB, et al. Anterior regions of the neck. In: Janfaza P, Nadol JB Jr, Galla RJ, et al, editors. Surgical anatomy of the head and neck. First Havard University Press Edition. Hagerstown, MA, USA: Lippincott Williams & Wilkins; 2001. p. 630–74.
11. Gray H, Standring S, Anhand N, editors. Gray's anatomy: the anatomical basis of clinical practice. 42nd edition. Elsevier; 2021.
12. Zakowski M, Vallejo MC. Chapter:1 Functional anatomy of the airway. In: Hagberg and benumof's airway management. 5th edition. Elsevier; 2023. p. 2–20.
13. Flynn W, Vickerton P. Anatomy, Head and Neck, Larynx Cartilage. In: StatPearls. StatPearls Publishing; 2022. Available at: http://www.ncbi.nlm.nih.gov/books/NBK553185/. Accessed February 5, 2023.
14. Suárez-Quintanilla J, Fernández Cabrera A, Sharma S. Anatomy, Head and Neck, Larynx. In: StatPearls. StatPearls Publishing; 2022. Available at: http://www.ncbi.nlm.nih.gov/books/NBK538202/. Accessed February 12, 2023.
15. Woodson GE. Upper airway anatomy and function. In: Byron J, editor. Bailey head & neck surgery-otolaryngology. 3rd edition. Lippincott William & Wilkins; 2001. p. 480–3.
16. Soriano RM, Winters R, Gupta V. Anatomy, Head and Neck, Larynx Nerves. In: StatPearls. StatPearls Publishing; 2022. http://www.ncbi.nlm.nih.gov/books/NBK557742/. Accessed February 12, 2023.
17. Culp JM, Patel G. Recurrent Laryngeal Nerve Injury. In: StatPearls. StatPearls Publishing; 2022. http://www.ncbi.nlm.nih.gov/books/NBK560832/. Accessed February 12, 2023.
18. Levine RJ, Sanders AB, LaMear WR. Bilateral vocal cord paralysis following blunt trauma to the neck. Ann Emerg Med 1995;25(2):253–5.
19. Malvi A, Jain S. Laryngeal trauma, its types, and management. Cureus 2022; 14(10):e29877.
20. Reza Nouraei SA, Sandhu GS. Chapter: 66 Laryngeal and esophageal trauma. In: Cummings otolaryngology: head and neck surgery. 7th edition. Elsevier Inc; 2021. p. 939–51.
21. Kim JD, Shuler FD, Mo B, et al. Traumatic laryngeal fracture in a collegiate basketball player. Sports Health 2013;5(3):273–5.
22. Yen PT, Lee HY, Tsai MH, et al. Clinical analysis of external laryngeal trauma. J Laryngol Otol 1994;108(3):221–5.
23. Butler APM, O'Rourke AKM, Wood BPM, et al. Acute External laryngeal trauma: experience with 112 patients. Ann Otol Rhinol Laryngol 2005;114(5):361–8.

24. Moonsamy P, Sachdeva UM, Morse CR. Management of laryngotracheal trauma. Ann Cardiothorac Surg 2018;7(2):210–6.

25. Wang AA, Feng AL, Rao V, et al. Clinical, radiologic, and endolaryngeal findings in laryngeal fractures: a 15-year case series. OTO Open 2022;6(1). https://doi.org/10.1177/2473974X221080164. 2473974X221080164.

26. Shi J, Uyeda JW, Duran-Mendicuti A, et al. Multidetector CT of laryngeal injuries: principles of injury recognition. Radiogr Rev Publ Radiol Soc N Am Inc 2019; 39(3):879–92.

27. Becker M, Leuchter I, Platon A, et al. Imaging of laryngeal trauma. Eur J Radiol 2014;83(1):142–54.

28. Corry M, Keyes C, Page D. Reviving freedom house. how the storied ambulance company has been reborn. JEMS J Emerg Med Serv 2013;38(3):70–5.

29. Liao CH, Huang JF, Chen SW, et al. Impact of deferred surgical intervention on the outcome of external laryngeal trauma. Ann Thorac Surg 2014;98(2):477–83.

30. Bell RB, Verschueren DS, Dierks EJ. Management of laryngeal trauma. Oral Maxillofacial Surg Clin N Am 2008;20(3):415–30.

31. On SW, Cho SW, Byun SH, et al. Bioabsorbable osteofixation materials for maxillofacial bone surgery: a review on polymers and magnesium-based materials. Biomedicines 2020;8(9):300.

32. Shires CB, Preston T, Thompson J. Pediatric laryngeal trauma: a case series at a tertiary children's hospital. Int J Pediatr Otorhinolaryngol 2011;75(3):401–8.

33. Sidell D, Mendelsohn AH, Shapiro NL, et al. Management and outcomes of laryngeal injuries in the pediatric population. Ann Otol Rhinol Laryngol 2011;120(12): 787–95.

34. Kurien M, Zachariah N. External laryngotracheal trauma in children. Int J Pediatr Otorhinolaryngol 1999;49(2):115–9.

Temporal Bone Trauma

James Dixon Johns, MD[a,b], Corinne Pittman, MD[a,b],
Selena E. Briggs, MD, PhD, MBA[a,b],*

KEYWORDS

- Temporal bone • Penetrating • Blunt • Trauma • Fracture • Complications

KEY POINTS

- Temporal bone fractures most commonly result from blunt trauma to the skull, although penetrating injuries more often result in significant complications.
- High-resolution computed tomography remains the gold standard for initial diagnosis of temporal bone trauma, and temporal bone fractures are frequently classified as "otic-capsule sparing" versus "otic-capsule violating" to characterize the risk stratification of these fractures.
- Hearing loss is the most common complication of temporal bone fractures; other potential complications include cranial nerve injury, cerebrospinal fluid leak, meningitis, vertigo, and vascular and vestibular complications.
- There remains a lack of universal guidelines regarding the management of temporal bone temporal bone trauma and their sequelae; further studies are needed in order to determine optimal risk stratification and optimal interventions regarding these patients.

INTRODUCTION

The paired temporal bones represent an important area of study as they form portions of the lateral skull base and house several critical structures, including the external, middle, and inner ear, multiple cranial nerves (CNs), as well as important vascular structures, including the internal carotid artery (ICA) and internal jugular vein (IJV). Trauma to the temporal bone may pose potentially deleterious sequelae owing to the intimate association of these vital structures as well as a conduit for further insult extending intracranially. The temporal bone encompasses the otic capsule, often considered the densest bone in the human body. Because of the significant force associated with temporal bone fractures, patients often present with other critical injuries that may delay diagnosis of temporal bone fractures. Injuries to the temporal bone may be overlooked during the initial trauma evaluation owing to severity of

a Department of Otolaryngology–Head and Neck Surgery, MedStar Georgetown University Hospital, Gorman Building, 1st Floor, 3800 Reservoir Road NW, Washington DC 20007, USA;
b Department of Otolaryngology–Head and Neck Surgery, MedStar Washington Hospital Center, 106 Irving Street Northwest, Suite 2700, Washington, DC 20010, USA
* Corresponding author. MedStar Washington Hospital Center, Department of Otolaryngology, 106 Irving Street Northwest, Suite 2700, Washington, DC 20010.
E-mail address: Selena.Briggs@medstar.net

Otolaryngol Clin N Am 56 (2023) 1055–1067
https://doi.org/10.1016/j.otc.2023.05.010
0030-6665/23/© 2023 Elsevier Inc. All rights reserved.

concomitant, critical comorbidities. The reported incidence of temporal bone trauma varies widely in the literature. This review highlights the current best evidence guiding the management of temporal bone trauma that has evolved the understanding of this important pathologic condition.

ANATOMY

The temporal bone comprises 4 bony partitions that each possess unique features (**Fig. 1**). The squamous segment encompasses the lateral aspect of the cranial vault and articulates with the sphenoid, frontal, and parietal bones at the pterion, the land-mark for the location of the middle meningeal artery.[2] The tympanic segment encom-passes the bony external auditory canal (EAC) and the middle ear cleft, which houses ossicles, tympanic segment of the facial nerve, and other vascular structures. The pneumatized mastoid segment of the temporal bone communicates with the middle ear via the aditus ad antrum and houses the vertical segment of the facial nerve that exits the temporal bone via the stylomastoid foramen. The petrous pyramid is located medially and contains the dense otic capsule the carotid canal, Meckel cave of the trigeminal nerve, and Dorello canal of the abducens nerve.[3]

EPIDEMIOLOGY

According to the Centers for Disease Control and Prevention, there are approximately 1.7 million traumatic head injuries in the United States annually. Of patients with trau-matic head injuries, approximately 4% experience skull fractures, and 14% to 22% of those are temporal bone fractures.[4] The prevalence of temporal bone fractures varies widely in the literature but is estimated to be approximately 3% of all trauma patients.[5]

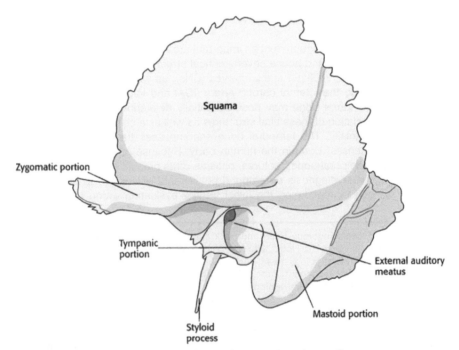

Fig. 1. Anatomy of temporal bone (adapted from Patel et al., 2010[1]).

These fractures may occur in any age group but most commonly occur in the second to fourth decades of life (70%) with a 3:1 female predominance.[6] Most temporal bones fractures are unilateral (80% of patients) with no preponderance for right versus left temporal bones.[6]

CAUSE

Temporal bone fractures most commonly result from blunt trauma to the skull. In the adult population, motor vehicle accidents represent the most frequent cause (55%), with mechanical falls (25%), industrial accidents (15%), and assault (4%) as other possible mechanisms. In contrast, the pediatric population experiences a higher proportion of temporal bone trauma resulting from mechanical falls (60%) compared with motor vehicle accidents (30%) (**Fig. 2**).[7]

CLASSIFICATION SYSTEMS

Classification schemes of temporal bone fractures have evolved over time. Early cadaveric studies by Gurdjian and Lissner[8] attempted to determine fracture patterns of the temporal bone based on anatomic orientation of the fracture lines in relation to the long axis of the petrous ridge (**Fig. 3**). This original scheme described fracture patterns as "longitudinal," "transverse," and "mixed," with early literature estimating approximately 90% of temporal bone fractures are longitudinal, 10% transverse, and 8% mixed. More recent literature reports variable rates of these fracture patterns in real-life experience compared with the original cadaveric studies.[9–11] Longitudinal fractures, which parallel the long axis of the petrous bone, include the EAC, resulting in conductive hearing loss (CHL) through tympanic membrane perforation and ossicular disruption. Transverse fractures, perpendicular to the long axis of petrous bone, result from trauma applied to the occipital bone with a fracture line extending through the internal auditory canal and otic capsule, resulting in sensorineural hearing loss (SNHL) and greater risk of facial nerve injury.[11]

These initial attempts at classification schemes set a foundation for other newer systems that prioritize the involvement of the petrous bone and otic capsule, which are better correlated with clinical symptoms and otologic outcomes. Dahiya and colleagues[10] proposed a modified classification system based primarily on otic-capsule–sparing versus otic-capsule–violating fracture lines. This system allows the provider to better understand the risk stratification of these fractures. Although otic-capsule–violating fractures represent 2.5% to 5.6% of temporal bone fractures, there is a two times greater risk of facial nerve paralysis, and higher rates of associated

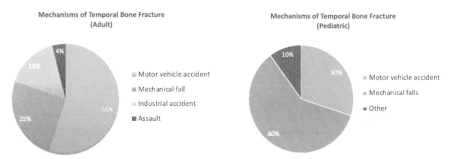

Fig. 2. Mechanisms of temporal bone fractures (adapted from Brown et al., 2023[7]).

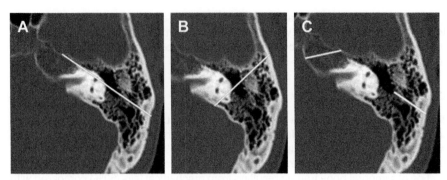

Fig. 3. Temporal bone fractures. Original classification system: longitudinal temporal bone fractures (*A*), transverse temporal bone fractures (*B*), mixed temporal bone fractures (*C*). Modified classification system: otic-capsule–violating fractures (*A, B*), otic-capsule–sparing fracture (*C*). The *white lines* depict the orientation of the fracture line upon which the origical classification system is based.

cerebrospinal fluid (CSF) leak (4 times) and severe SNHL (7 times) compared with otic-capsule–sparing fractures.[6,10] Approximately 95% of temporal bone fractures are otic-capsule sparing.[6] Other published classifications systems also aim to relate patient symptoms and outcomes with the type of fracture patterns, offering a means of prognosis in the acute and long-term follow-up phases of care.[11,12]

PENETRATING TRAUMA

Penetrating injuries of the temporal bone, including gunshot injuries and stab wounds, are far less common than blunt injuries, but are more likely to result in complications. Gunshot wounds to the head involve the temporal bone in approximately 20% to 50% of cases.[13,14] Firearms have a range of associated velocities with low-velocity firearms (eg, shotgun) ranging from 90 to 120 m/s to high-velocity firearms (eg, military-grade firearms) propelling at greater than 610 m/s.[15,16] Gunshot wounds typically involve the midface, entering beneath the orbit or in the periauricular region, and sparing the otic capsule, as it sits in a high-density bone that deflects the path of a projectile. The presence of shrapnel does not require debridement (**Fig. 4**). Rather, surgical management

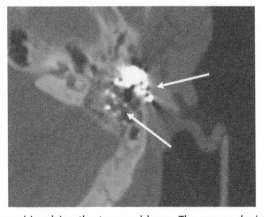

Fig. 4. Gunshot wound involving the temporal bone. The *arrows* depicts shrapnel (bullet fragments) lodged within the mastoid.

is governed by associated injury or associated risk of complication (ie, damage to the EAC, CSF leak, facial nerve injury).

For patients who survive a temporal bone gunshot wound, facial nerve injury occurs in up to 50% with most patients presenting with complete facial paralysis.[15,17] Because of the presence of dispersed shrapnel, it is often challenging to localize the precise site of facial nerve injury by computed tomography (CT) scan.[15,17] Patients may undergo operative management, including facial nerve decompression and repair, if necessary. However, in many cases, some degree of facial nerve dysfunction persists. **Fig. 5** depicts the CT scan from a patient who sustained a penetrating stab wound to the temporal bone, severing the labyrinthine segment of the facial nerve. Operative management via the middle fossa approach was used with decompression and cable grafting using the greater auricular nerve. At 1-year follow-up, the patient's facial function was graded a House-Brackmann 4.

Another complication of a gunshot injury to the temporal bone includes CSF leaks.[15,18] Surgical intervention for a CSF leak is indicated in cases of a persistent leak that fails to resolve spontaneously or by conservative management with a lumbar drain.[15,18] With extensive tegmen defects, encephaloceles may form.[16,19] Major vascular injuries are also a possible outcome of a gunshot wound injury to the temporal bone and typically require surgical or endovascular treatment to achieve hemostasis. Long-term injury to the EAC may result in canal stenosis. Over time, cholesteatoma (more commonly from canal stenosis and less commonly theoretically from skin implantation) may develop.

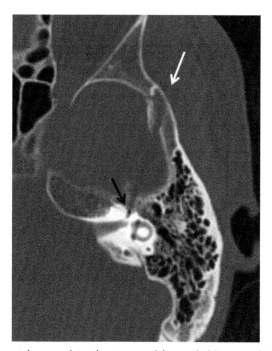

Fig. 5. Penetrating stab wound to the temporal bone. (*white arrow*) Point of calvarial. (*black arrow*) Location of injury at the first genu.

EVALUATION AND DIAGNOSIS
History and Physical Examination

Following assessment of the primary trauma examination and stabilization of the patient, a thorough head and neck examination should be performed. Important considerations for the clinical examination involve accurate documentation of facial nerve function and thorough inspection of the ear. Although the CN examination may be limited owing to concomitant morbidity or sedation, the timing and extent of facial nerve weakness may guide treatment recommendations and are important in the initial examination. Careful inspection and documentation of the ear involve evaluating for lacerations, exposed cartilage, auricular hematoma, postauricular ecchymosis (Battle sign), bloody or clear (CSF) otorrhea, tympanic perforation, and hemotympanum. It is recommended to avoid suctioning or insufflation of the ear canal in the event of cerumen or blood obscuring view of tympanic membrane owing to the risk of CSF otorrhea.[20]

Radiographic Evaluation

High-resolution (CT dedicated to the temporal bone and internal auditory canal remains the gold standard for initial diagnosis and evaluation of temporal bone fractures. CT angiography is superior to noncontrast CT when vascular injury is suspected.[7,21]

Audiologic Evaluation

In the acute setting, patients may be evaluated with whispered voice or tuning forks examination. Thorough audiometric evaluation, including audiometry and acoustic reflex testing, may be performed at initial evaluation and at least 2 months following injury following resolution of hemotympanum to assess for type and severity of hearing loss.[7,20]

Electrodiagnostic Evaluation

Although there is no consensus on electrodiagnostic testing following temporal bone trauma with facial nerve palsy, the guidelines established by Esslen and Fisch[22] and Gantz and colleagues[23] for idiopathic facial nerve palsy may be considered. Patients may undergo electroneurography (ENOG) and electromyography (EMG) to assist in prognosticating the extent and likelihood of facial nerve function recovery. ENOG may be used within 3 to 14 days following injury to assess facial nerve motor responses to supramaximal stimulus from the affected side, with more than 90% reduction compared with the contralateral side, indicating a poorer prognosis of adequate recovery.[23] EMG may be used to assess for the absence of end motor action potentials or development of fibrillation potentials that may portend poorer prognosis for facial nerve recovery.[23]

COMPLICATIONS
Hearing Loss

Hearing loss is one of the most common sequelae of temporal bone trauma. A patient may experience CHL, SNHL, or mixed hearing loss (MHL), depending on the location and extent of the injury to the temporal bone. Otic-capsule–sparing temporal bone fractures more commonly result with CHL through a variety of possible mechanisms based on the fracture pattern, including conductive losses via tympanic membrane perforation, hemotympanum, or ossicular chain disruption. Given that otic-capsule–sparing fractures encompass most of these injuries, it is not unexpected that CHL comprise the predominant pattern of postfracture hearing loss with incidences reported at 26% to 57%.[24,25] Transient CHL may be encountered owing to hemotympanum, which typically improves over time,[26] although permanent CHL results from ossicular chain disruption, which may occur in approximately 20% of patients.[27] Of ossicular chain disruptions (**Fig. 6**), the most common injuries include incudostapedial subluxation (82%), incus dislocation (57%), and fracture of the stapes crura (30%).[28] Middle ear surgery may be indicated with evidence of ossicular chain disruption or persistent CHL over 2 months postinjury without identifiable cause.[20]

Conversely, otic-capsule–violating temporal bone fractures more commonly result in an SNHL (14% to 23%) or MHL (20% to 55%)[29,30] owing to perilymphatic fistula, damage to hair cells or cochlear nerve, disruption of cochlear blood supply, and labyrinthine concussion. A recent study by Park and colleagues[26] demonstrated that otic-capsule–violating temporal bone fractures involving the cochlea or vestibule were significantly more likely to result in SNHL compared with otic-capsule–violating fractures involving the semicircular canal or other otic-capsule–sparing fractures. Although air conduction thresholds typically improved after 30 weeks, the bone conduction thresholds did not significantly improve despite age of patient or use of steroids.[26] For this reason, there have been recent studies regarding the efficacy of cochlear implantation in posttraumatic SNHL, although traumatic and anatomic limitations must be considered, including the risk of development of labyrinthitis ossificans with delayed procedures posttrauma.[31,32]

Cranial Nerve Injury

There are multiple CNs that course within or in close proximity to the temporal bone that are vulnerable to injury during temporal bone trauma. CN V and CN VI may be injured during trauma to the petrous portion of the temporal bone as they pass along Meckel cave and Dorello canal, respectively. CN VII and VIII enter the temporal bone via the internal auditory canal and synapse with the structures within the otic capsule, posing high risk for injury during otic-capsule–violating fractures. Fractures extending to the foramen magnum or jugular foramen may present risks to the delicate neurovascular structures that pass through them, including CN X and XI. These intricate relationships highlight the importance of a thorough clinical correlation with the

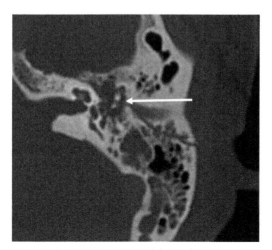

Fig. 6. Transverse, otic-capsule–sparing temporal bone fracture with ossicular disruption. Axial CT scan depicting separation of the incudomalleolar joint (*arrow*).

radiographic evaluation, as the extent of nerve injuries may be difficult to predict from imaging alone.

Because of the circuitous route through the temporal bone, CN VII is the most commonly injured CN in temporal bone fractures with most injuries occurring along the first genu (perigeniculate segment) of the nerve followed by the tympanic segment.[26,33,34] Prior studies suggest that CN VII injuries occur in 7% to 34% of patients, with CN VII palsies nearly twice as common in otic-capsule–violating fractures compared with otic-capsule–sparing fractures (33.3% vs 15.8%).[10,26] Following CN VII injury, complete recovery is less common, whereas most patients improve to House-Brackmann grade 3 or better (93%–100%).[26,30]

Mechanisms of CN injury range from neuropraxia from neural edema to complete neurotmesis.[35] For this reason, one of the fundamental components of initial evaluation is a thorough clinical examination, as timing and extent of CN palsy may assist the decision making of optimal management strategies. CN VII injuries may be categorized as "acute" (within 1 day) or "delayed" (beyond 1 day) and "complete" or 'incomplete." CN VII that are "delayed" portend a better prognosis for recovery and are often managed less aggressively with either observation, steroids, antivirals, or combinations thereof.[6,20,36] Many providers consider the 2013 American Academy of Otolaryngology-Head and Neck Surgery guidelines regarding management of Bell palsy, which strongly advocate for the use of oral corticosteroids within 72 hours of onset with or without antivirals, with no firm recommendation on the role of surgical intervention.[37]

Surgical facial nerve decompression involves removing bony barriers overlying the nerve to prevent restriction during neural edema. Consistent improvement following facial nerve decompression may be limited with complete recovery of CN VII rates in approximately 23% of cases, whereas complication rates may range from 0% to 15%.[21,36,38,39] Prior studies by Gantz and colleagues[23] proposed criteria for the role of surgical intervention in idiopathic facial paralysis with improvement in function for select patients based on ENOG reduction greater than 90% in amplitude with absent voluntary EMG activity 3 to 14 days after onset. Despite numerous studies, there remains no consensus guidelines on the management of these injuries in traumatic temporal bone fractures.[37] Consistent improvement following facial nerve decompression may be limited with complete recovery of CN VII rates in approximately 23% of cases, whereas complication rates may range from 0% to 15%.[21,36,38,39]

Cerebrospinal Fluid Leak/Perilymphatic Fistula

CSF leaks represent an important complication of temporal bone fractures and may present as clear otorrhea or rhinorrhea if the tympanic membrane remains intact. It is estimated to occur in approximately 17% of temporal bone fractures, and the location of leakage may vary by fracture pattern.[6] In otic-capsule–sparing fractures, the leak is thought to more commonly occur through the tegmen tympani or tegmen mastoideum.[20] In otic-capsule–violating fractures, the CSF may leak from the posterior fossa into the middle ear via the otic capsule. Because of the minimal bony remodeling of the otic capsule in adulthood, these fractures may heal with variable scar formation that may pose extended risk of continued communication and possible meningitis.[20]

For this reason, it is an important consideration in the clinical examination to examine for evidence of CSF leak. Common complaints include headache and clear drainage from ear or nose that worsens when bearing down or leaning forward. Laboratory testing for CSF includes identification of beta-2 transferrin, which is an isoform of transferrin that is specific for CSF, perilymph, and aqueous humor.[40] CSF leakage is typically managed conservatively with bedrest, head of bed elevation, and precautions to reduce intracranial pressure, including the use of stool softeners and sinus precautions. It has been estimated that 57% to 85% of leaks spontaneously resolve within 1 week with conservative management, and there are no consensus guidelines advocating for the use of antibiotic prophylaxis in uncomplicated CSF leaks.[20,41,42] When CSF fistulae persist beyond 7 to 10 days, operative closure may be indicated to reduce the risk of meningitis.[20]

Meningitis

Although CSF leaks present a relatively low risk of persistent CSF fistula, intracranial spread of infection and resultant meningitis remain important, potentially life-threatening, complications of temporal bone fractures. Increased duration of CSF fistula is thought to be a significant risk factor for the development of meningitis.[43,44] The most common pathogens associated with meningitis in CSF fistula are *Pneumococcus*, followed by *Streptococcus*, and *Haemophilus influenzae*.[45–47] A meta-analysis by Brodie[43,48] demonstrated that meningitis occurred in 8.7% of patients with posttraumatic CSF fistulae, and that this risk was reduced to 2.1% with the use of prophylactic antibiotics. Conversely, the Cochrane Database meta-analysis from 2006 and 2011 revealed no significant difference in the rate of meningitis in antibiotic therapy group versus control.[49,50] Despite this, there remains no consensus within the literature regarding the use of prophylactic antibiotics.

Vascular Complication

Because of the proximity of multiple critical structures with the temporal bone, vascular complications are an additional consideration with temporal bone trauma. As discussed, vascular structures that may be injured during temporal bone fractures include the temporal bone, the intratemporal ICA, middle meningeal artery, IJV/jugular bulb, and sigmoid sinus. Potential vascular complications are vast and range from laceration of vessel with resultant hemorrhage, aneurysm, dissection, fistula, impingement, or resultant thrombosis. Intratemporal ICA injury remains among the most feared life-threatening vascular complications, although this is rare owing to the relatively thick bone covering the carotid canal.[20] If ICA injury suspected, the patient should undergo urgent packing of EAC and further imaging to assess for the need for acute intervention. One study of pediatric temporal bone fractures estimated rates of venous thrombosis and intracranial arterial dissection to be approximately 0.4% for both complications.[51]

Vestibular Dysfunction

Vertigo is a relatively common complication following temporal bone trauma. The most common transient vertiginous condition following head trauma is benign paroxysmal positional vertigo, with most cases resolving within 6 to 8 weeks following trauma.[20,52] Patients with temporal bone fractures may experience more severe forms of vertigo owing to insults to neurovascular contributions to the vestibular system, including superior semicircular canal dehiscence or perilymphatic fistula.[53] Labyrinthine dehiscence and perilymphatic fistula may be encountered following temporal bone trauma, with patients complaining of strain- or pressure-induced vertigo. Another possible cause of vertigo following temporal bone trauma involves fracture-associated posttraumatic endolymphatic hydrops.[54] This rare clinical entity is thought to result from traumatic obstruction of endolymphatic flow through the vestibular aqueduct and endolymphatic sac at the operculum, presenting with a triad of symptoms mimicking Ménière syndrome, including low-frequency SNHL, aural fullness, and vertigo.[54]

Vestibular testing may support diagnosis in addition to radiographic evaluation and include cervical or ocular vestibular–evoked myogenic potentials, Fistula (Hennebert) test, or Tullio testing.[55] Conservative treatment involves avoidance of instigating factors, carbonic anhydrase inhibitors, and diuretics, as these processes are often refractory to common vestibular suppressant medical management.[55] In refractory cases, surgical intervention may be indicated to address anatomic contributions of vertigo.

FUTURE DIRECTIONS

Despite the increasing literature on the diagnosis and management of temporal bone trauma, there are limited consensus guidelines regarding this topic. Further studies are needed in order to determine optimal risk stratification and optimal interventions regarding these patients.

SUMMARY

Temporal bone trauma remains an important clinical entity. Because of the high-force requirements of injury, patients may also have significant concomitant injury that may preclude early identification of temporal bone trauma and sequelae. Despite this, there are many important clinical considerations of temporal bone trauma that must be considered. Because of the numerous critical structures that may be involved in temporal bone trauma, it remains of paramount importance for thorough evaluation of management of these sequelae.

Although the temporal bone encompasses the otic capsule, often considered the densest bone in the human body, tremendous force is required to fracture the temporal bone. Because of the significant force associated with temporal bone fracture, patients often present with other critical injuries that may delay diagnosis of temporal bone fractures.

CLINICS CARE POINTS

- Temporal bone fractures most commonly result from blunt trauma to the skull, although penetrating injuries more often result in significant complications.

- High-resolution computed tomography (CT) remains the gold standard for initial diagnosis of temporal bone trauma, and temporal bone fractures are frequently classified as "otic-capsule sparing" versus "otic-capsule violating" to characterize the risk stratification of these fractures.

- Hearing loss is the most common complication of temporal bone fractures; other potential omplications include cranial nerve (CN) injury, cerebrospinal fluid (CSF) leak, meningitis, vertigo, vascular and vestibular complications.

- There remains a lack of universal guidelines regarding the management of temporal bone temporal bone trauma and their sequelae; further studies are needed in order to determine optimal risk stratification and optimal interventions regarding these patients.

DISCLOSURE

No disclosures.

REFERENCES

1. Patel A, Groppo E. Management of temporal bone trauma. Craniomaxillofac Trauma Reconstr 2010;3(2):105–13.

2. Muche A. Positions and Types of Pterion in Adult Human Skulls: A Preliminary Study. Ethiop J Health Sci 2021;31(4):875–84.

3. Nayak S. Segmental anatomy of the temporal bone. Semin Ultrasound CT MR 2001;22(3):184–218.

4. Roozenbeek B, Maas AI, Menon DK. Changing patterns in the epidemiology of traumatic brain injury. Nat Rev Neurol 2013;9(4):231–6.

5. Zayas JO, Feliciano YZ, Hadley CR, et al. Temporal bone trauma and the role of multidetector CT in the emergency department. Radiographics 2011;31(6): 1741–55.

6. Brodie HA, Thompson TC. Management of complications from 820 temporal bone fractures. Am J Otol 1997;18(2):188–97.

7. Brown J, Hohman MH, Shermetaro C. Facial nerve intratemporal trauma. StatPearls. StatPearls Publishing Copyright © 2023. Treasure Island, FL: StatPearls Publishing LLC; 2023.

8. Gurdjian ES, Lissner HR. Deformations of the skull in head injury studied by the stresscoat technique, quantitative determinations. Surg Gynecol Obstet 1946;83: 219–33.

9. Tos M. Course of and sequelae to 248 petrosal fractures. Acta Otolaryngol 1973; 75(4):353–4.

10. Dahiya R, Keller JD, Litofsky NS, et al. Temporal bone fractures: otic capsule sparing versus otic capsule violating clinical and radiographic considerations. J Trauma 1999;47(6):1079–83.

11. Kang HM, Kim MG, Boo SH, et al. Comparison of the clinical relevance of traditional and new classification systems of temporal bone fractures. Eur Arch Oto-Rhino-Laryngol 2012;269(8):1893–9.

12. Rafferty MA, Mc Conn Walsh R, Walsh MA. A comparison of temporal bone fracture classification systems. Clin Otolaryngol 2006;31(4):287–91.

13. Hagan WE, Tabb HG, Cox RH, et al. Gunshot injury to the temporal bone: an analysis of thirty-five cases. Laryngoscope 1979;89(8):1258–72.

14. Haberkamp TJ, McFadden E, Khafagy Y, et al. Gunshot injuries of the temporal bone. Laryngoscope 1995;105(10):1053–7.

15. Backous DD, Minor LB, Niparko JK. Trauma to the external auditory canal and temporal bone. Otolaryngol Clin North Am 1996;29(5):853–66.

16. Kilty S, Murphy PG. Penetrating temporal bone trauma. J Trauma 2009;66(3): E39–41.

17. Bento RF, de Brito RV. Gunshot wounds to the facial nerve. Otol Neurotol 2004; 25(6):1009–13.

18. Kahn JB, Stewart MG, Diaz-Marchan PJ. Acute temporal bone trauma: utility of high-resolution computed tomography. Am J Otol 2000;21(5):743–52.

19. Harris JP, Anterasian G, Hoi SU, et al. Management of carotid artery transection resulting from a stab wound to the ear. Laryngoscope 1985;95(7 Pt 1):782–5.

20. Diaz RC, Cervenka B, Brodie HA. Treatment of Temporal Bone Fractures. J Neurol Surg B Skull Base 2016;77(5):419–29.

21. Nash JJ, Friedland DR, Boorsma KJ, et al. Management and outcomes of facial paralysis from intratemporal blunt trauma: a systematic review. Laryngoscope 2010;120(7):1397–404.

22. Esslen E, Fisch U. Localization of nerve damage in idiopathic facial paresis and the question of decompression. Schweiz Med Wochenschr 1971;101(11):386–7. Zur Lokalisation der Nervenschädigung bei der idiopathischen Fazialisparese und Zur Frage der Dekompression.

23. Gantz BJ, Rubinstein JT, Gidley P, et al. Surgical management of Bell's palsy. Laryngoscope 1999;109(8):1177–88.

24. Ghorayeb BY, Yeakley JW. Temporal bone fractures: longitudinal or oblique? The case for oblique temporal bone fractures. Laryngoscope 1992;102(2):129–34.

25. Nosan DK, Benecke JE Jr, Murr AH. Current perspective on temporal bone trauma. Otolaryngol Head Neck Surg 1997;117(1):67–71.

26. Park E, Chang YS, Kim BJ, et al. Improved Prediction of Hearing Loss after Temporal Bone Fracture by Applying a Detailed Classification for Otic Capsule-Violating Fracture: A Wide Scope Analysis with Large Case Series. Otol Neurotol 2023;44(2):153–60.

27. Yoganandan N, Pintar FA, Sances A Jr, et al. Biomechanics of skull fracture. J Neurotrauma 1995;12(4):659–68.

28. Hough JV, Stuart WD. Middle ear injuries in skull trauma. Laryngoscope 1968; 78(6):899–937.

29. Ishman SL, Friedland DR. Temporal bone fractures: traditional classification and clinical relevance. Laryngoscope 2004;114(10):1734–41.

30. Darrouzet V, Duclos JY, Liguoro D, et al. Management of facial paralysis resulting from temporal bone fractures: Our experience in 115 cases. Otolaryngol Head Neck Surg 2001;125(1):77–84.

31. Greenberg SL, Shipp D, Lin VY, et al. Cochlear implantation in patients with bilateral severe sensorineural hearing loss after major blunt head trauma. Otol Neurotol 2011;32(1):48–54.

32. Medina M, Di Lella F, Di Trapani G, et al. Cochlear implantation versus auditory brainstem implantation in bilateral total deafness after head trauma: personal experience and review of the literature. Otol Neurotol 2014;35(2):260–70.

33. Yanagihara N. Transmastoid decompression of the facial nerve in temporal bone fracture. Otolaryngol Head Neck Surg 1982;90(5):616–21.

34. Lambert PR, Brackmann DE. Facial paralysis in longitudinal temporal bone fractures: a review of 26 cases. Laryngoscope 1984;94(8):1022–6.

35. Chang CY, Cass SP. Management of facial nerve injury due to temporal bone trauma. Am J Otol 1999;20(1):96–114.

36. Wamkpah NS, Kallogjeri D, Snyder-Warwick AK, et al. Incidence and Management of Facial Paralysis After Skull Base Trauma, an Administrative Database Study. Otol Neurotol 2022;43(10):e1180–6.

37. Baugh RF, Basura GJ, Ishii LE, et al. Clinical practice guideline: Bell's palsy. Otolaryngol Head Neck Surg 2013;149(3 Suppl):S1–27.

38. Bento RF, Pirana S, Sweet R, et al. The role of the middle fossa approach in the management of traumatic facial paralysis. Ear Nose Throat J 2004;83(12): 817–23.

39. Sanuş GZ, Tanriöver N, Tanriverdi T, et al. Late decompression in patients with acute facial nerve paralysis after temporal bone fracture. Turk Neurosurg 2007; 17(1):7–12.

40. Meurman OH, Irjala K, Suonpää J, et al. A new method for the identification of cerebrospinal fluid leakage. Acta Otolaryngol 1979;87(3–4):366–9.

41. Lewin W. Cerebrospinal fluid rhinorrhea in nonmissile head injuries. Clin Neurosurg 1964;12:237–52.

42. Frazee RC, Mucha P Jr, Farnell MB, et al. Meningitis after basilar skull fracture. Does antibiotic prophylaxis help? Postgrad Med 1988;83(5):267–8, 273-4.

43. Leech PJ, Paterson A. Conservative and operative management for cerebrospinal-fluid leakage after closed head injury. Lancet 1973;1(7811): 1013–6.

44. Spetzler RF, Wilson CB. Management of recurrent CSF rhinorrhea of the middle and posterior fossa. J Neurosurg 1978;49(3):393–7.
45. MacGee EE, Cauthen JC, Brackett CE. Meningitis following acute traumatic cerebrospinal fluid fistula. J Neurosurg 1970;33(3):312–6.
46. Appelbaum E. Meningitis following trauma to the head and face. JAMA 1960;173: 1818–22.
47. Kaufman BA, Tunkel AR, Pryor JC, et al. Meningitis in the neurosurgical patient. Infect Dis Clin North Am 1990;4(4):677–701.
48. Brodie HA. Prophylactic antibiotics for posttraumatic cerebrospinal fluid fistulae. A meta-analysis. Arch Otolaryngol Head Neck Surg 1997;123(7):749–52.
49. Ratilal B, Costa J, Sampaio C. Antibiotic prophylaxis for preventing meningitis in patients with basilar skull fractures. Cochrane Database Syst Rev 2006;(1): Cd004884.
50. Ratilal BO, Costa J, Sampaio C, et al. Antibiotic prophylaxis for preventing meningitis in patients with basilar skull fractures. Cochrane Database Syst Rev 2011;(8):Cd004884.
51. Adepoju A, Adamo MA. Posttraumatic complications in pediatric skull fracture: dural sinus thrombosis, arterial dissection, and cerebrospinal fluid leakage. J Neurosurg Pediatr 2017;20(6):598–603.
52. Schuknecht HF. Mechanism of inner ear injury from blows to the head. Ann Otol Rhinol Laryngol 1969;78(2):253–62.
53. Peng KA, Ahmed S, Yang I, et al. Temporal bone fracture causing superior semicircular canal dehiscence. Case Rep Otolaryngol 2014;2014:817291.
54. Bächinger D, Goosmann MM, Schuknecht B, et al. Clinical Imaging Findings of Vestibular Aqueduct Trauma in a Patient With Posttraumatic Meniere's Syndrome. Front Neurol 2019;10:431.
55. Gianoli GJ. Post-concussive Dizziness: A Review and Clinical Approach to the Patient. Front Neurol 2021;12:718318.

Perioperative Management of Patients with Craniomaxillofacial Trauma

Tzu-Hsuan Cheng, MD[a], Matthew Mendelsohn, MD[b],
Radhika Patel, MD[c], Samrat Worah, MD[a], Sydney C. Butts, MD[b,d],*

KEYWORDS

- Substance abuse • Postoperative pain management • Urine toxicology screen
- Facial fracture complications • Difficult airway management

KEY POINTS

- Have adequate instrumentation to temporize the airway in facial fracture patients who may present with oral cavity or oropharyngeal edema.
- Understand how to interpret the urine toxicology screen and distinguish between acute intoxication and chronic morbidity from substance abuse.
- Respect the challenges of perioperative analgesia management in patients with facial fractures. Multimodal analgesia and collaboration with pain management physicians are central to patient satisfaction.

INTRODUCTION

The perioperative management of patients with craniomaxillofacial trauma involves multidisciplinary collaboration among emergency department physicians, facial trauma surgeons, anesthesiology, nursing, and other clinicians for patients with polytrauma. Facial trauma severity determines the acuity of intervention and although some patients require immediate operative reconstruction, many others can be scheduled on an urgent basis shortly after the injury has been diagnosed.[1,2] Guidelines for timing of treatment recommend therapeutic windows within 1 to 10 days after the injury depending on the facial subsite.[3–5] These guidelines balance the need to

---

[a] Department of Anesthesiology, State University of New York-Downstate Health Sciences University, 450 Clarkson Avenue, Brooklyn, NY 11203, USA; [b] Department of Otolaryngology, State University of New York-Downstate Health Sciences University, 450 Clarkson Avenue, Brooklyn, NY 11203, USA; [c] State University of New York-Downstate Health Sciences University, 450 Clarkson Avenue, Brooklyn, NY 11203, USA; [d] Division of Facial Plastic Surgery, Department of Otolaryngology, Kings County Hospital Center, Brooklyn, NY, USA
* Corresponding author. SUNY Downstate Health Sciences University, Department of Otolaryngology, 450 Clarkson Avenue, Brooklyn, NY 11203.
E-mail address: sydney.butts@downstate.edu

Otolaryngol Clin N Am 56 (2023) 1069–1078
https://doi.org/10.1016/j.otc.2023.05.015
0030-6665/23/© 2023 Elsevier Inc. All rights reserved.

restore form and function before the onset of scar contracture, infection, or other complications of delayed treatment with operating room resource and personnel availability.[2,3,6]

After facial injuries have been diagnosed and stabilized, a management plan must be developed that addresses several areas including perioperative pain management and surgical risk assessment by the anesthesia team. Evidence-based guidance in these areas has evolved over the last several years. The multimodal/opioid-sparing analgesia approaches that have emerged as best practices for postoperative pain management in the last decade are a direct response to the opioid epidemic.[7,8]

Close communication between the anesthesiology and surgical teams is essential in the perioperative management of patients with facial fractures. The assessment and management of the airway is a joint undertaking and should be reviewed in the context of sources of potential airway obstruction that is associated with facial fractures.

The dangers that place people at risk for facial trauma are heightened by the use of legal or illicit substances.[9,10] The use of substances may impact not only the acute trauma presentation but chronic use may result in comorbidities that affect the patient's perioperative risk stratification.[10-12] We describe the perioperative risks for patients who test positive for illicit drugs at initial trauma evaluation, and review the current evidence about how the use of other substances impacts perioperative management by the anesthesia and surgical teams.

INITIAL PATIENT ASSESSMENT

The history gathering for the patient presenting with otolaryngologic trauma has been reviewed in the articles in this issue focusing on specific head and neck regions. Key points to emphasize include details of the mechanism of trauma, which determines the degree of soft tissue and bony disruption. Degrees of blood loss and injuries to deeper structures are more likely to occur with penetrating trauma compared with blunt injuries. Head and neck trauma patients may also develop airway compromise secondary to several mechanisms including penetrating or blunt trauma of the neck that involve vascular structures, muscles, or the larynx.

The standard history gathering to determine comorbidities is central, because surgery for head and neck trauma patients either needs to be scheduled emergently or urgently. This may pose some challenges in attempts to confirm medications and may not allow time to hold or reverse anticoagulation. Social habits including smoking, alcohol intake or abuse, and use of any controlled or illicit substances must be documented. Conversations during history gathering must be detailed, given the legalization of substances, which patients may not consider dangerous including marijuana, vaping, herbals, and narcotics that are prescribed or obtained by other means. The occupational history of patients who are victims of trauma is also important if the injury occurred at the workplace and because the patient will need guidance about time out of work or away from athletics for patients who are students in school.[13]

PHYSICAL EXAMINATION

The initial evaluation of a head and neck trauma patient involves implementation of Advanced Trauma Life Support protocols and stabilization of life-threatening injuries. Concomitant injuries of the cervical spine must be ruled out along with head trauma in consultation with the emergency physicians, trauma surgeons, and the neurosurgical team. Associated head trauma resulting in intracranial bleeding warrants high priority in the management hierarchy but other types of head trauma has also received greater recognition as a comorbid injury among facial trauma patients.[14,15] Concussions associated with fractures of the mandible and midface require attention and assessment in the immediate and subacute trauma period.[14,15] It may not be possible to rule out cervical spine injury before emergent intubation, thus cervical spine immobilization by a second individual should be performed via manual in-line stabilization while the airway is managed (**Fig. 1**). Manual in-line stabilization can worsen the laryngoscopic view, resulting in the clinician applying greater pressure that can transmit to the cervical spine or take longer causing failure to secure the airway.

Patients with mandible fractures may present with trismus, defined as an interincisal mouth opening of less than 4 cm making the intraoral examination more challenging and management of the airway more difficult (**Fig. 2**). Trismus associated with facial fractures is usually secondary to splinting from pain or edema of the muscles of mastication. Often, with induction of anesthesia, visualization during laryngoscopy is adequate but preparation with instrumentation to enhance the view of the airway is the safest approach during intubation of patients with facial fractures. Other scenarios may result in airway compromise requiring intervention before definitive management of any fractures. Impingement on the airway may result from a hematoma of the tongue or floor of mouth secondary to a comminuted fracture of the mandible. Glossoptosis and narrowing of the oropharyngeal airway can develop in patients with bilateral condylar fractures, which leads to retrognathia (**Fig. 3**).[16] It is essential that clinicians ensure the immediate availability of adequate airway equipment including nasal and oral airways, laryngoscope blades, video-assisted intubating devices, a flexible bronchoscope, multiple sizes of endotracheal tubes, a bougie, laryngeal mask airway (LMA), and a cricothyroidotomy kit.

Standard laboratory tests are ordered based on the patient's history and comorbidities. For many trauma patients, it is routine that urine toxicology and blood alcohol levels are ordered given the high rates of substance abuse associated with these injuries.[9,10,12] It is important to understand the physiologic impact of certain substances and anticipate adjustments in the anesthesia protocols for patients who test positive during screening examinations, which is reviewed in the next section.

COCAINE

Cocaine produces prolonged adrenergic stimulation by blocking the presynaptic uptake of sympathomimetic neurotransmitters, including norepinephrine, serotonin, and

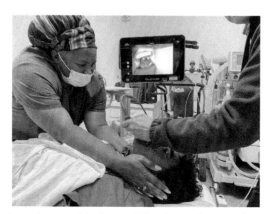

Fig. 1. Demonstration of manual in-line stabilization technique during intubation on a mannequin.

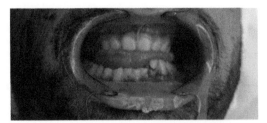

Fig. 2. Trismus. The patient has a comminuted mandible fracture with interincisal opening approximately 2 cm. Maximal interincisal opening should be no less than 4 cm.

dopamine.[17,18] Its use can lead to multiple cardiovascular comorbidities, including hypertension, tachycardia, prolonged QT interval, coronary vasospasm, myocardial infarction, aortic dissection, and stroke.[19,20] Some pulmonary complications, such as aspiration pneumonia, noncardiogenic pulmonary edema, and pulmonary hypertension, have been associated with chronic cocaine use.[21]

Cocaine has a half-life of 45 to 90 minutes and is metabolized by plasma and liver esterase. The conventional urine toxicology test for cocaine detects the presence of its inactive metabolites for up to a week after cocaine use. A 1-week cocaine abstinence period before elective surgery under general anesthesia has been recommended.[21] However, recent evidence has shown that general anesthesia for cocaine users who are asymptomatic is not associated with a higher risk of cardiac morbidity.[11,22,23] Thus, a urine toxicology result positive for cocaine may not reflect an absolute contraindication to proceeding with a surgical procedure. The cancellation rate with elective

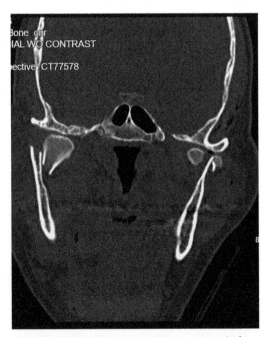

Fig. 3. Bilateral condylar fractures. Airway narrowing can result from posterior displacement of the mandible and narrowing of the airway.

surgery for cocaine users remains high. Elkassabany and colleagues[24] found only 10.6% anesthesia departments have formal perioperative guidelines for cocaine-positive patients, which may explain high cancellation rates and points to the need for perioperative management guidelines or practice advisory for cocaine-abusing patients.

The preoperative assessment must determine the timing of the last dose of cocaine use and the patient's history of cocaine use. Cardiac evaluation may be necessary, including an electrocardiogram and echocardiogram. Patients should be counseled on the potential risks of perioperative cocaine use. If the patient is acutely intoxicated with cocaine, then general anesthesia is not recommended for elective cases.[25]

Ryb and Cooper[26] looked at outcomes of cocaine-positive trauma patients undergoing surgery on the first day of admission. Cocaine-positive patients had no statistically significant difference in the rate of death, or length of stay, compared with their counterparts.[26]

MARIJUANA

Therapeutic and recreational use of cannabinoids have significantly increased in the United States within the last two decades because of regulatory changes and its therapeutic uses. Cannabinoids remain the most used illicit recreational drug in the United States, according to the 2019 National Survey on Drug Use and Health. Perioperative cannabis increases perioperative risks given its interaction with anesthetic medications and postoperative analgesics. The dose-dependent cognitive function impairment associated with cannabinoids can make informed consent challenging for acutely intoxicated patients. According to a systematic review, recovery of cognitive function may take up to 5 to 7 hours after inhaling delta-9-tetrahydrocannabinol (Δ9-THC). A dose-dependent increase in heart rate, systolic blood pressure, and cardiac output is caused by the activation of the sympathetic nervous system. With the higher cannabis dosage and chronic cannabis use, parasympathetic tone increases, which is manifested as postural hypotension and bradycardia. A recent cohort study has shown cannabinoids increased the risk of perioperative myocardial infarction because of increased myocardial oxygen demand. The adjusted odds of postoperative myocardial infarction was 1.88 (95% confidence interval, 1.31–2.69)[27] times higher for patients with a reported active cannabis use disorder compared with those without.[28–30] Synthetic cannabis smoking is also associated with pulmonary embolism,.[31,32] Chronic cannabinoid use may worsen postoperative pain and precipitate postoperative hyperalgesia.[33–35] McAfee and colleagues[36] found cannabis users report worse pain, more centralized pain symptoms, and greater sleep disturbances versus cannabis nonusers on the day of surgery.

A consensus guideline published by the American Society of Regional Anesthesia in 2023 addressed the perioperative challenges that arise from managing patients taking cannabis and cannabinoids. Universal toxicology screening for cannabinoids is not recommended because of insufficient evidence. Regarding whether to stop cannabinoids perioperatively, although recent reviews recommended cannabinoid cessation 72 hours before surgery,[37,38] abrupt cessation of cannabinoids-based medication perioperatively may cause adverse effects including cannabis withdrawal syndrome marked by seizures, tachycardia, chest pain, or palpitations.[39]

Levine and colleagues[40] evaluated the prevalence of marijuana use among trauma patients before and after legalization of medical marijuana and found marijuana use among trauma patients was four-fold higher compared with the general population.

Sokoya and colleagues[41] looked at patterns of facial trauma before and after legalization of marijuana, reporting increased rates of maxillary and skull base fracture; rates of mandibular, Le Fort, zygomaticomaxillary, nasal bone, and orbital fractures were not increased.

METHAMPHETAMINE

Amphetamines are the third most widely abused class of drugs in the United States. They also are used medically as treatments for attention-deficit/hyperactivity disorder, exogenous obesity, and narcolepsy.

Methamphetamine is a sympathomimetic drug that causes the release of endogenous dopamine, norepinephrine, and serotonin. Stimulation from methamphetamine causes 2 to 10 times more dopamine to be released from endogenous stores than the natural response. It reaches its peak plasma level 2.5 to 4 hours after smoking, with a plasma half-life of 10 hours. At low doses (5–30 mg) methamphetamine causes increased arousal, restlessness, and hyperthermia. Prolonged muscle contractions can lead to severe acidosis, rhabdomyolysis, hyperkalemia, and sudden cardiac arrest.[42] Other cardiovascular effects include hypertension, pulmonary arterial hypertension, and coronary vasospasm. Serious cardiovascular side effects, such as methamphetamine-associated cardiomyopathy, myocardial infarction, aortic dissection, ischemic stroke, and sudden death, are reported at high doses.[43,44]

Patients who present to the operating room with a positive urine drug screen for amphetamines within 2 days of surgery are at increased risk of hemodynamic instability and require a higher rate of pressors despite being administered lower doses of anesthetic medications.[45] Constant stimulation of adrenergic receptors in the central and peripheral nervous system results in receptor downregulation and catecholamine depletion, eliminating the body's sympathetic response to hypotension.[46] Direct-acting vasopressors should be used to treat hypotension or bradycardia. The administration of succinylcholine is contraindicated because of increased risk of rhabdomyolysis, hyperkalemia, and impaired cardiac conduction.

CIGARETTE SMOKING

Chronic exposure to cigarette smoke produces profound changes in physiology because of its constituents, nicotine and carbon monoxide. Smoking is a known risk factor for cardiovascular diseases, such as coronary artery and peripheral vascular disease. It potentiates myocardial work by increasing heart rate, blood pressure, and myocardial contractility via elevation in sympathetic tone and circulating catecholamines. Oxygen delivery is impaired by carboxyhemoglobin, levels of which may exceed 10% in smokers.[47] Perioperative pulmonary, wound healing, cardiovascular, and other complications are more likely in patients who have continued smoking up until the time of surgery.

POSTOPERATIVE PAIN MANAGEMENT

The management of perioperative pain in trauma patients is challenging, especially in the setting of prior substance abuse.[48] Physician-related factors add to the complexity of decision making. Principles of pain management that could be learned during medical school or residency may not be emphasized in surgical curricula.[48] Evidence that specifically addresses recommendations for postoperative pain management in facial trauma patients are few compared with other areas of surgery. These have increased over the last 10 to 15 years in parallel with calls for opioid-sparing postoperative analgesia protocols generally[8,49] and evidence-based facial trauma guidelines specifically.[5,50]

Adequate pain management for trauma patients requires identification of adequate analgesics to relieve moderate to severe pain, regularly reassessing patients and reevaluating their pain management regimen, and weighing the risk and benefits of adverse effects of pain medications.[50] The central role that opioid analgesics have traditionally had for postoperative pain control has been called into question. The availability of a wider selection of agents allows options that may provide better efficacy, a safer side effect profile, or both.[8] Public and governmental level concerns about addiction to narcotics have resulted in marked increases in prescriber monitoring.[49]

Multimodal analgesia has been shown to decrease morphine use in adult trauma patients.[51,52] Nonsteroidal anti-inflammatory drugs (NSAIDs) are an important nonopioid component of the multimodal analgesic approach. Levels of postoperative pain are reported to be highest for mandibular fractures compared with fractures of the midface (when comparing isolated rather than multiple fractures).[53] Ibuprofen and acetaminophen/paracetamol have all been shown to have efficacy in the postoperative setting for patients with mandible fractures.[50,54] Several studies have reported diminished need for opioids with the prescription of nonselective NSAIDS[55–57] and cyclooxygenase-2 inhibitors.[54] Few adverse effects were reported with the use of NSAIDS. Although patient follow-up in these studies was typically short (24 hours after surgery) no reports of postoperative bleeding were noted, which is one of the leading concerns with NSAIDs use.[54–57] Another approach to accomplish multimodal postoperative analgesia for facial fracture patients is the injection of long-acting local anesthetics to block branches of the trigeminal nerve. Blockade of the inferior alveolar nerve or the mental nerve with bupivacaine has been described resulting in a decreased need for opioids and an increased time between emergence from anesthesia and the request for additional analgesia.[58,59]

SUMMARY

Complications in facial fracture management, both surgical and from general anesthesia, are minimized or avoided by adhering to recommendations from current evidence-based publications. Surgeons and anesthesiologists must work together at numerous points and make joint decisions especially where airway and pain management challenges may arise.

CLINICS CARE POINTS

- Urine toxicology screening is frequently ordered for trauma patients. More comprehensive recommendations are needed to guide the preoperative work-up based on test results of patients to avoid unnecessary surgical delays or cancellations.
- Opioid-sparing postoperative analgesia approaches offer adequate pain control to facial trauma patients and minimizes adverse effects associated with narcotics.

DISCLOSURE

The authors declare that there are no relevant commercial or financial interests that relate to the research discussed in this article.

REFERENCES

1. Hsieh TY, Funamura JL, Dedhia R, et al. Risk Factors Associated With Complications After Treatment of Mandible Fractures. JAMA Facial Plast Surg 2019;21(3):213–20.
2. Dougherty WM, Christophel JJ, Park SS. Evidence-based medicine in facial trauma. Facial Plast Surg Clin North Am 2017;25(4):629–43.
3. Morrow BT, Samson TD, Schubert W, et al. Evidence-based medicine: Mandible fractures. Plast Reconstr Surg 2014;134(6):1381–90.
4. Bregman JA, Vakharia KT, Idowu OO, et al. Outpatient Surgical Management of Orbital Blowout Fractures. Craniomaxillofac Trauma Reconstr 2019;12(3):205–10.
5. Nasser M, Pandis N, Fleming PS, et al. Interventions for the management of mandibular fractures. Cochrane Database Syst Rev 2013;7:Cd006087.
6. Alpert B, Kushner GM, Tiwana PS. Contemporary management of infected mandibular fractures. Craniomaxillofac Trauma Reconstr 2008;1(1):25–9.
7. Helmerhorst GT, Teunis T, Janssen SJ, Ring D. An epidemic of the use, misuse and overdose of opioids and deaths due to overdose, in the United States and Canada: is Europe next? Bone Joint J 2017;99:856–64.
8. Anne S., Mims J.W., Tunkel D.E., et al., Clinical Practice Guideline: Opioid Prescribing for Analgesia After Common Otolaryngology Operations. Otolaryngol Head Neck Surg. 2021;164(2_suppl):S1-S42.
9. Chang SL, Patel V, Giltner J, et al. The relationship between ocular trauma and substance abuse in emergency department patients. Am J Emerg Med 2017;35(11):1734–7.
10. McAllister P, Jenner S, Laverick S. Toxicology screening in oral and maxillofacial trauma patients. Br J Oral Maxillofac Surg 2013;51(8):773–8.
11. Saggese NP, Chang C, Cardo VA. Perioperative management for the cocaine-positive patient undergoing elective surgery under general anesthesia. J Oral Maxillofac Surg 2019;77(5):894–5.
12. Carrigan TD, Field H, Illingworth RN, et al. Toxicological screening in trauma. J Accid Emerg Med 2000;17(1):33–7.
13. Borgna SC, Klein K, Harvey LE, et al. Factors affecting return to work following facial trauma. Plast Reconstr Surg 2013;132(6):1525–30.
14. Sobin L, Kopp R, Walsh R, et al. Incidence of Concussion in Patients With Isolated Mandible Fractures. JAMA Facial Plast Surg 2016;18(1):15–8.
15. McCarty JC, Kiwanuka E, Gadkaree S, et al. Traumatic Brain Injury in Trauma Patients With Isolated Facial Fractures. J Craniofac Surg 2020;31(5):1182–5.
16. Mooney S, Gulati RD, Yusupov S, et al. Mandibular Condylar Fractures. Facial Plast Surg Clin North Am 2022;30(1):85–98.
17. Cunningham KA, Callahan PM. Monoamine reuptake inhibitors enhance the discriminative state induced by cocaine in the rat. Psychopharmacology (Berl) 1991;104(2):177–80.
18. Benowitz NL. Clinical pharmacology and toxicology of cocaine. Pharmacol Toxicol 1993;72(1):3–12.
19. Baxter JL, Alexandrov AW. Utility of cocaine drug screens to predict safe delivery of general anesthesia for elective surgical patients. AANA J (Am Assoc Nurse Anesth) 2012;80(4 Suppl):S33–6.
20. Granite EL, Farber NJ, Adler P. Parameters for treatment of cocaine-positive patients. J Oral Maxillofac Surg 2007;65(10):1984–9.
21. Beaulieu P. Anesthetic implications of recreational drug use. Can J Anaesth 2017;64(12):1236–64.

22. Moon TS, Pak TJ, Kim A, et al. A Positive Cocaine Urine Toxicology Test and the Effect on Intraoperative Hemodynamics Under General Anesthesia. Anesth Analg 2021;132(2):308–16.
23. Hill GE, Ogunnaike BO, Johnson ER. General anaesthesia for the cocaine abusing patient. Is it safe? Br J Anaesth 2006;97(5):654–7.
24. Elkassabany N, Speck RM, Oslin D, et al. Preoperative screening and case cancellation in cocaine-abusing veterans scheduled for elective surgery. Anesthesiol Res Pract 2013;2013:149892. https://doi.org/10.1155/2013/149892.
25. Richards JR, Le JK. Cocaine toxicity. Treasure Island (FL: StatPearls Publishing Copyright © 2023, StatPearls Publishing LLC; 2023. StatPearls.
26. Ryb GE, Cooper C. Outcomes of cocaine-positive trauma patients undergoing surgery on the first day after admission. J Trauma 2008;65(4):809–12.
27. Goel A, McGuinness B, Jivraj NK, et al. Cannabis Use Disorder and Perioperative Outcomes in Major Elective Surgeries: A Retrospective Cohort Analysis. Anesthesiology 2020;132(4):625–35.
28. Mallat A, Roberson J, Brock-Utne JG. Preoperative marijuana inhalation: an airway concern. Can J Anaesth 1996;43(7):691–3.
29. Pertwee RG. Neuropharmacology and therapeutic potential of cannabinoids. Addict Biol 2000;5(1):37–46.
30. Guarisco JL, Cheney ML, LeJeune FE Jr, Reed HT. Isolated uvulitis secondary to marijuana use. Laryngoscope 1988;98(12):1309–12.
31. Raheemullah A, Laurence TN. Repeated thrombosis after synthetic cannabinoid use. J Emerg Med 2016;51(5):540–3.
32. Yırgın G, Ateş İ, Katipoğlu B, et al. Pulmonary embolism due to synthetic cannabinoid use: Case report. Turk Kardiyol Dern Ars 2018;46(5):411–3.
33. Wallace M, Schulteis G, Atkinson JH, et al. Dose-dependent effects of smoked cannabis on capsaicin-induced pain and hyperalgesia in healthy volunteers. Anesthesiology 2007;107(5):785–96.
34. Hill KP, Palastro MD, Johnson B, et al. Cannabis and Pain: A Clinical Review. Cannabis Cannabinoid Res 2017;2(1):96–104.
35. Dupriest K, Rogers K, Thakur B, et al. Postoperative Pain Management Is Influenced by Previous Cannabis Use in Neurosurgical Patients. J Neurosci Nurs 2021;53(2):87–91.
36. McAfee J, Boehnke KF, Moser SM, et al. Perioperative cannabis use: a longitudinal study of associated clinical characteristics and surgical outcomes. Reg Anesth Pain Med 2021;46(2):137–44.
37. Echeverria-Villalobos M, Todeschini AB, Stoicea N, et al. Perioperative care of cannabis users: A comprehensive review of pharmacological and anesthetic considerations. J Clin Anesth 2019;57:41–9.
38. Huson HB, Granados TM, Rasko Y. Surgical considerations of marijuana use in elective procedures. Heliyon 2018;4(9):e00779.
39. Laudanski K, Wain J. Considerations for cannabinoids in perioperative care by anesthesiologists. J Clin Med 2022;11(3). https://www.mdpi.com/2077-0383/11/3/558.
40. Levine M., Jontz A., Dabrowski P., et al., Prevalence of marijuana use among trauma patients before and after legalization of medical marijuana: the Arizona experience, *Subst Abus*, 42 (3), 2021, 366–371.
41. Sokoya M., Eagles J., Okland T., et al., Patterns of facial trauma before and after legalization of marijuana in Denver, Colorado: a joint study between two Denver hospitals, *Am J Emerg Med*, 36 (5), 2018, 780–783.

42. Sperling LS, Horowitz JL. Methamphetamine-induced choreoathetosis and rhab-domyolysis. Ann Intern Med 1994;121(12):986.

43. Huang MC, Yang SY, Lin SK, et al. Risk of Cardiovascular Diseases and Stroke Events in Methamphetamine Users: A 10-Year Follow-Up Study. J Clin Psychiatry 2016;77(10):1396–403.

44. Schwarzbach V, Lenk K, Laufs U. Methamphetamine-related cardiovascular dis-eases. ESC Heart Fail 2020;7(2):407–14.

45. Safdari KM, Converse C, Dong F, et al. Hemodynamic Effects of Methamphet-amine and General Anesthesia. Anesthesiol Res Pract 2022;2022:7542311.

46. Johnston RR, Way WL, Miller RD. Alteration of anesthetic requirement by amphet-amine. Anesthesiology 1972;36(4):357–63.

47. Gilbert DD. Chemical analyses as validators in smoking cessation programs. J Behav Med 1993;16(3):295–308.

48. Lapidus JB, Santosa KB, Skolnick GB, et al. Opioid Prescribing and Use Patterns in Postsurgical Facial Trauma Patients. Plast Reconstr Surg 2020;145(3):780–9.

49. Curtis C, Scarcella J, Viscardi C, et al. Reduction of Opioid Prescriptions in Maxil-lofacial Trauma Following North Carolina STOP Act." Craniomaxillofac Trauma. Reconstr 2021;14(3):231–5.

50. Butts SC, Floyd E, Lai E, et al. Reporting of Postoperative Pain Management Pro-tocols in Randomized Clinical Trials of Mandibular Fracture Repair: A Systematic Review. JAMA Facial Plast Surg 2015;17(6):440–8.

51. Drahos AL, Scott AM, Johns TJ, et al. Multimodal Analgesia and Decreased Opioid Use in Adult Trauma Patients. Am Surg 2020;86(8):950–4.

52. Burton SW, Riojas C, Gesin G, et al. Multimodal analgesia reduces opioid require-ments in trauma patients with rib fractures. J Trauma Acute Care Surg 2022;92(3): 588–96.

53. Peisker A, Meissner W, Raschke GF, et al. Quality of Postoperative Pain Manage-ment After Maxillofacial Fracture Repair. J Craniofac Surg 2018;29(3):720–5.

54. Goswami D, Sardar A, Baidya DK, et al. Comparative Evaluation of Two Doses of Etoricoxib (90 mg and 120 mg) as Pre-Emptive Analgesic for Post-Operative Pain Relief in Mandibular Fracture Surgery Under General Anaesthesia: A Prospective, Randomised, Double-Blinded, Placebo-Controlled Trial. Turk J Anaesthesiol Re-anim 2020;48(1):24–30.

55. Eftekharian HR, Ilkhani Pak H. Effect of intravenous ketorolac on postoperative pain in mandibular fracture surgery; a randomized, double-blind, placebo-controlled trial. Bull Emerg Trauma 2017;5(1):13–7.

56. Jain AD, Vsm R, Ksn SB, et al. A Comparative Assessment of Postoperative Anal-gesic Efficacy of Lornoxicam versus Tramadol after Open Reduction and Internal Fixation of Mandibular Fractures. Craniomaxillofac Trauma Reconstr 2017;10(3): 171–4.

57. Nezafati S, Khiavi RK, Mirinejhad SS, et al. Comparison of Pain Relief from Different Intravenous Doses of Ketorolac after Reduction of Mandibular Fractures. J Clin Diagn Res 2017;11(9). c06–pc10.

58. Mesgarzadeh AH, Afsari H, Pourkhamne S, et al. Efficacy of bilateral mental nerve block with bupivacaine for postoperative pain control in mandibular para-symphysis fractures. J Dent Res Dent Clin Dent Prospects 2014;8(3):172–5.

59. Sawhney C, Agrawal P, Soni KD. Post operative pain relief through intermittent mandibular nerve block. Natl J Maxillofac Surg 2011;2(1):80–1.

Approaches to the Maxillofacial Skeleton
Application of Standard and Minimally Invasive Techniques

Abigail B. Thomas, MD*, Sachin S. Pawar, MD

KEYWORDS

- Trauma • Maxillofacial • Endoscopic fracture repair • Minimally invasive
- Frontal sinus • Orbit • Midface • Mandible

KEY POINTS

- Thorough knowledge of facial anatomy, indications, surgical techniques, and potential complications will facilitate decision-making for approaches to repair facial fractures.
- A combination of approaches can often be used to provide optimal access to facial fractures.
- Endoscopic approaches and other minimally invasive approaches may be used in select patients for management of frontal sinus, orbital and subcondylar/condylar fractures.

INTRODUCTION

Adequate exposure of the maxillofacial skeleton is crucial for the assessment and repair of traumatic injuries. Direct exposure allows for expeditious and safe surgery. Exposure on the face is complicated by the need for esthetic considerations and avoidance of important structural landmarks. There is a variety of approaches and techniques that can be used to achieve exposure under these conditions. We will review the standard, more commonly used approaches by facial region, as well as discuss more novel and minimally invasive techniques.

FRONTAL SINUS

Frontal sinus fractures account for 5% to 15% of all facial fractures.[1] Management of frontal sinus fractures is highly variable, leading to the advent of treatment algorithms to help with decision on approach. Repair depends on involvement of anterior or

Department of Otolaryngology and Communication Sciences, Medical College of Wisconsin, 8701 Watertown Plank Road, Milwaukee, WI 53226, USA
* Corresponding author.
E-mail address: abthomas@mcw.edu

Otolaryngol Clin N Am 56 (2023) 1079–1088
https://doi.org/10.1016/j.otc.2023.05.003
0030-6665/23/Published by Elsevier Inc.

posterior tables, frontal sinus outflow tract (FSOT), skull base, and the severity of the fractures. Minimally displaced, isolated anterior table fractures can often be observed if there is no concern for contour deformity.[1]

Existing Lacerations

Facial fractures are often associated with overlying lacerations, which can be used as direct access to the facial bones. In the frontal/forehead region, lacerations can be extended for use, then closed within the horizontal frontalis and vertical glabellar resting skin tension lines.

Coronal/Bitemporal Approach

The coronal/bitemporal approach allows for exposure of the upper two-thirds of the craniomaxillofacial (CMF) skeleton, including the orbits and zygoma. The incision is hidden behind the hairline and a perichondrial flap can be raised for use in frontal sinus repairs but there is the risk of alopecia, numbness, and injury to the facial nerve.[2] This remains the approach of choice for comminuted, depressed anterior table fractures and posterior table fractures requiring obliteration or cranialization.[1]

Minimally Invasive Transcutaneous Approaches

The use of suprabrow and subbrow incisions can provide a more direct approach to smaller, less complex anterior table fractures, decreasing operative time while still allowing for adequate reduction.[3,4] The suprabrow approach is placed at the lateral superior border of the eyebrow, similar to a direct browlift incision, allowing for direct visualization of fractures and ease of reduction and fixation. Care is taken to preserve the supratrochlear and supraorbital nerves.[3] The subbrow approach has been described to provide similar ease of access and favorable cosmetic results.[4] The incision is placed at the medial inferior aspect of the eyebrow and dissection is taken down to the superior orbital rim.

Endoscopic

Endoscopic brow approaches can provide adequate exposure for isolated injuries of the anterior table while minimizing incisions.[5–7] This approach should be avoided for greatly depressed and displaced fractures, as well as those with high hairlines or thinning hair. Combined with the use of percutaneous incisions for screw placement, implants can be placed and fixed to camouflage frontal sinus irregularity.[8] Endonasal endoscopic approaches offer the ability to treat concomitant FSOT injuries, anterior table fractures, and some posterior table injuries.[9–11] The ability to assess and address mucosal and sinus health is also of importance in treatment of frontal sinus injuries, which can be done concomitantly with endoscopic approaches.[10] With advances in endoscopic sinus surgery, there has been a shift toward early observation of patients with unclear FSOT injuries, with the ability to repair in a delayed fashion if functional sinus concerns develop.[1,9,12]

The biggest drawback to endoscopic approaches for all traumas remains the steep learning curve and need for earlier training to ensure safe repairs.[13] Superior and laterally based fractures can also be hard to access with endoscopic equipment but the use of a brow incision and trephine with the endoscope can improve accessibility.[14]

NASO-ORBITO-ETHMOID COMPLEX

Naso-orbito-ethmoid (NOE) fractures can be difficult to access and repair. Need for repair mostly depends on the status of the medial canthal tendon (MCT). If the MCT is separated from the maxilla, correction of telecanthus is required. A bicoronal approach is the historical gold-standard but midfacial degloving (MFD) can also be used.[5,15] MFD involves maxillary sublabial incisions with midface elevation to the extent of the fractures. Complications of MFD include nasal disruption leading to changed cosmesis and nasal airway obstruction.[15] Given the frequency that NOE fractures are accompanying other midface fractures, use of local lacerations or necessary orbital approaches can often provide adequate exposure without additional incisions.[15] A direct glabellar approach can be used, although it is best in older patients with existing horizontal rhytids, to camouflage the incision.

ORBIT

Orbital floor and medial wall are the most common orbital injuries seen in adults.[16] Many orbital fractures can be monitored and managed nonoperatively, depending on intact vision, signs of entrapment, extent of fracture/orbital volume change, and cosmesis. There are a myriad of ways to enter and repair the orbit, often depending on which wall is fractured.[2]

Transconjunctival

Transconjunctival approaches are commonly used for orbital floors and are favored for their concealed incision and reduced risk of postoperative ectopion.[2,14] This approach can be preseptal (avoids risk of herniated fat) or postseptal (faster rim exposure, avoids eyelid dissection).[2] By extending a transconjunctival incision medially, it is made into a transcaruncular approach, allowing for medial wall access. For increased lateral wall exposure, a swinging eyelid approach is made by extending a transconjunctival incision with the use of lateral canthotomy and cantholysis. This increases the exposure to the lateral orbit and zygoma while minimizing the risk of laceration or stretching (leading to lagophthalmos) of the lower eyelid with retraction. Care must be taken at closure for lateral canthal reapproximation but studies have shown there is minimal to no difference in cosmetic outcomes when lateral extension is used.[17,18]

Transcutaneous

Transcutaneous approaches give similar orbital floor access and have lower risk of ectropion with healing but visible scars and retraction of the lower eyelid are a risk.[2,19] These incisions can be made subciliary, subtarsal, or at the infraorbital rim. A subciliary incision can be extended laterally to allow for lateral rim access. The superior orbital rim can be accessed through the previously discussed bicoronal incision or brow incisions also used for frontal sinuses. A more direct upper blepharoplasty approach offers extended lateral orbital rim visualization, with a cosmetically appealing incision.[2]

Endoscopic

Endoscopy can also be a useful adjunct in the repair of orbital fractures. Medial orbital wall injuries can be easily accessed via endonasal endoscopic approach with or without a small transconjunctival incision for the placement of implants if needed. This is a familiar approach for otolaryngologists with sinus surgery training and can reduce operative time and complications for patients.[20–22]

For orbital floor visualization and repair, endoscopy is especially useful.[14,23,24] Transmaxillary (via Caldwell-Luc) and transantral approaches have been described throughout the literature. If the orbital floor fracture is part of a zygomaticomaxillary complex (ZMC) fracture, the endoscope can be introduced through the maxillary sinus via a sublabial incision. For isolated orbital floor fractures, a Caldwell-Luc incision can be used.[14] Both of these approaches avoid manipulation of the eyelid and improve visualization for fracture management. A transorbital endoscopic approach has also been described, using a transconjunctival approach. Visualization was improved and with a similar complication profile to endonasal endoscopic orbital approaches.[25]

MAXILLA/ZYGOMA

Maxillary fractures are often classified via LeFort classification based on the buttress system. The midface has 3 vertical buttresses (nasomaxillary [NM], zygomaticomaxillary [ZM], and pterygomaxillary) and 3 horizontal buttresses (frontal bar/supraorbital rim; inferior orbital rim and zygomatic arch; and maxillary hard palate).[26] The surgical approach will vary depending on the fracture pattern and laterality of injuries. For simple fractures, a single approach can be used, whereas complex fractures will likely need multiple combined approaches. Superior midface traumas, involving the zygomatic arch or previously discussed orbit or NOE complex, may necessitate a bicoronal approach for access, or a combination of brow incisions, extended transcutaneous/transconjunctival orbital approaches, and percutaneous access.[26]

Transcutaneous

For extensive trauma requiring complete midfacial exposure, Weber-Fergusson incisions have historically been used. This transcutaneous approach follows the boundaries of facial subunits to hide the incision line but can still lead to extensive scarring and disfigurement. Transcutaneous approaches, such as lateral brow or lateral blepharoplasty incisions, can give direct access to the lateral orbital rim and zygomaticofrontal buttress.[27]

Intraoral

The intraoral and intranasal incisions of MFD may be necessary for complete lower midface exposure but the majority of maxillary and ZMC fractures can be adequately exposed via intraoral gingivobuccal incisions through a maxillary vestibular approach.[14,26] Intraoral approaches allow access to the ZM and NM buttresses and are also useful for ZMC fractures.[27]

Minimally Invasive

Isolated zygomatic arch fractures can be addressed indirectly through minimally invasive Gillies or Keen approaches. The Gillies approach uses a 2-cm incision in the temporal hairline and dissection down in a plane deep to the superficial layer of the deep temporal fascia to protect the overlying frontal branch of the facial nerve. Reduction is then achieved with the use of an elevator through this dissection plane with placement below the depressed zygomatic arch segment. The intraoral Keen approach uses a small incision in the lateral maxillary vestibule for the placement of an elevator below the zygomatic arch. This approach facilitates direct palpation with a finger to assess reduction of the arch.[28]

MANDIBLE

Mandibular trauma is extremely common and the mandible is the most commonly fractured facial bone requiring surgical repair.[16] The location and pattern of fractures will guide type of repair and approach. Historically, mandible fractures were often treated with "closed" approaches using various techniques of maxillomandibular fixation (MMF). However, with the advent of plating systems, the standard of care now typically involves open reduction and internal fixation (ORIF) through a variety of approaches.[2,14,16]

Intraoral

Most mandible fractures will require rigid plating through ORIF. ORIF can be performed through a transoral mandibular vestibular approach or a transfacial/transcervical approach.[2,16] The benefits of transoral approach are the obvious lack of facial scarring and decreased risk to facial and marginal mandibular nerve but can limit the surgeon's view and lead to poor reduction. The mandibular vestibular approach gives excellent access to symphyseal, parasymphyseal, and most body fractures, with the only real concern of protecting the mental nerve.[2] Placement of plates and screws on the posterior body and angle can be difficult through vestibular incisions, which can be alleviated with the use of a transbuccal trocar or angled screw drivers.

Transcutaneous

Transcutaneous approaches have the benefit of greater and direct visualization and often more accessibility for plate placement. The biggest risk is facial or marginal mandibular nerve injury, along with scarring and salivary gland/duct injury.[16,29] These approaches are often classified by their proximity to the nerve.

Although less commonly used, a transcervical approach via apron incision gives broad exposure to the entire mandible, akin to a bicoronal approach for large frontal fractures. This approach can be considered with severely comminuted fractures requiring broad exposure, patient with trismus, temporomandibular joint (TMJ) ankyloses, or atrophic mandibles.[30] The submental approach can be used to access symphyseal and parasymphyseal fractures. Although these fractures are usually accessed via vestibular intraoral incisions, highly comminuted fractures can be an indication for submental access. Overlying chin lacerations can also be incorporated into submental incisions.

Transcutaneous approaches are also used for ORIF of subcondylar and condylar fractures. Historically, MMF was the primary treatment due to poor accessibility to these fractures. In recent years, there has been more of a focus on open reduction to avoid weeks of closed stabilization and the potential for TMJ ankylosis.[16,29] Current indications for reduction include condylar displacement, lack of posterior molars, concomitant panfacial/midface fractures, and foreign body.[29] Subcondylar fractures are most often accessed through transcutaneous approaches; however, transoral endoscopic approaches have also been used as described below.

A preauricular approach places the incision in the preauricular crease above the main trunk of the facial nerve. It is useful for access to the condyle and upper subcondylar neck.[2] A submandibular, or Risdon, approach uses an incision at least 2 cm below the angle of the mandible, for marginal mandibular nerve protection, and parallel to the mandible or within a skin crease. It is useful for angle, ramus, and lower subcondylar neck fractures.[2] The retromandibular approach is the most direct approach to the ramus, condylar, and subcondylar region but also carries the high risk of facial nerve injury.[2] An anteroparotid transmasseteric approach is an alternative to the retromandibular approach that has shown more nerve protection. Incision is made preauricular in a parotidectomy fashion, then dissection is taken through the SMAS, over the parotid, then down through the masseter for direct access to the ramus.[31,32]

Table 1
Areas of access and limitations of maxillofacial skeleton approaches

	Approach	Access	Limitations
Frontal	Existing lacerations	Underlying bony fractures	Irregular access
	Coronal/bitemporal	Frontal sinus/forehead, zygoma/zygomatic arch, orbit (except floor), nasal bones	Large incision, alopecia, facial n. injury
	Endoscopic brow	Anterior table, nasal bones	Supratrochlear and supraorbital neurovascular injuries, visualization
	Endoscopic transnasal	FSOT, anterior and posterior table	Hard to access lateral injuries
NOE	Coronal/bitemporal	Frontal sinus/forehead, zygoma/zygomatic arch, orbit (except floor), nasal bones	Large incision, alopecia, facial n. injury
	Glabellar	Nasal bones, NOE	Poor cosmesis
Orbit	Transconjunctival—medial/transcaruncular	Orbital floor, infraorbital rim, medial wall	Eye trauma, entropion, lacrimal injury, anterior ethmoidal a. injury
	Transconjunctival—lateral/swinging eyelid	Orbital floor, infraorbital rim, lateral wall, zygomaticofrontal (ZF) buttress	Eye trauma, entropion, lagophthalmos, poor cosmesis
	Transcutaneous—subciliary/subtarsal	Orbital floor, infraorbital rim, zygoma	Eye trauma, ectropion, scarring
	Transcutaneous—lateral brow	ZF buttress, superolateral orbital rim	Alopecia, scarring, limited exposure
	Transcutaneous—upper bleph	ZF buttress, superolateral orbital rim (more than lateral brow)	Eye trauma, poor cosmesis
	Endoscopic transnasal	Medial orbital wall, orbital floor	Often in combo with external approach, limited access, need endoscopy experience
	Endoscopic transorbital	Medial orbital wall, orbital floor	Through an external incision, learning curve
Maxilla/Zygoma	Weber-Fergusson	Orbital floor, ZMC, maxilla, nasal bones	Large incision, poor cosmesis
	MFD	Bilateral nasal bones, nasal soft tissue/cartilage, infraorbital rim, zygoma	Nasal soft tissue/cartilage disruption, infraorbital n. injury
	Intraoral maxillary vestibular	Infraorbital rim, maxilla, ZM buttress, zygoma, lateral nasal bones	Infraorbital n. injury
	Temporal (Gillies)	Zygomatic arch	No fixation, superficial temporal a. or facial n. injury, scaring
	Transoral (Keen)	Zygomatic arch	No fixation

Region	Approach	Exposure	Complications
Mandible	Intraoral mandibular vestibular	Mandibular body, symphysis, angle	Difficult access to posterior angle/subcondylar, mental n. injury
	Transcervical	Mandibular symphysis, body, angle, ramus	Large incision; marginal mandibular n., facial a. and v. injury, scarring
	Submental	Symphysis, parasymphysis	Limited access
	Preauricular	Condylar head and neck, TMJ	Limited exposure; facial n., superficial temporal a. or v. injury; scarring
	Submandibular/Risdon	Posterior body, angle, ramus, subcondylar	Marginal mandibular n., facial a. or v. injury; scarring
	Retromandibular	Ramus, condyle	Facial n. or retromandibular v. injury
	Anteroparotid transmasseteric	Angle, ramus, condyle	Parotid injury, facial n. or greater auricular n. injury; scarring
	Endoscopic	Angle, ramus, condyle	Need experience/time to learn, poor visualization

Endoscopic

Endoscopic approaches are also used in mandible fractures for an improved visualization and reduced risk to nerves and facial scarring compared with transcutaneous approaches. The biggest limitations of endoscopy continue to be the steep learning curve and often long operative times, as well as the need for specialized equipment.[29,33] There are also complex fracture patterns that are not amenable to endoscopic reduction. Endoscopic approaches do not always mitigate the need for transcutaneous incisions, often requiring a transcutaneous trocar placement for drilling and screw placement. This limitation can be addressed with the advent of angled drills and screwdrivers, an example showing that continued improvement in technology and instrumentation will continue to improve treatment options for difficult mandible fractures.[29]

SUMMARY

There is a myriad of approaches to the maxillofacial skeleton for the management of facial fractures. Decisions regarding the approach depend on anatomic location of the fractures and extent, surgeon comfort, and goals for repair. Standard transcutaneous, larger exposure approaches are being replaced or augmented by minimally invasive techniques through smaller incisions, thanks in part to technology, such as endoscopic equipment and angled screwdrivers. These techniques are making difficult to treat areas, such as the frontal sinus, orbital wall and subcondylar mandible, more accessible and easier to manage while decreasing potential surgical risks and recovery time for the patient (**Table 1**).

CLINICS CARE POINTS

- Thorough knowledge of facial anatomy, indications, surgical techniques, and potential complications will facilitate decision-making for approaches to repair facial fractures.
- A combination of approaches can often be used to provide optimal access to facial fractures.
- Endoscopic approaches and other minimally invasive approaches may be used in select patients for the management of frontal sinus, orbital, and subcondylar/condylar fractures.

REFERENCES

1. Dedhia RD, Morisada MV, Tollefson TT, et al. Contemporary management of frontal sinus fractures. Curr Opin Otolaryngol Head Neck Surg 2019;27(4): 253–60.
2. Ellis IE, Zide MF. Surgical approaches to the facial skeleton. 3rd edition. Philadelphia: Wolters Kluwer; 2018.
3. Hahn HM, Lee YJ, Park MC, et al. Reduction of closed frontal sinus fractures through suprabrow approach. Arch Craniofacial Surg 2017;18(4):230–7.
4. Kim J, Choi H. A review of subbrow approach in the management of noncomplicated anterior table frontal sinus fracture. Arch Craniofacial Surg 2016; 17(4):186.
5. Pawar SS, Rhee JS. Frontal sinus and naso-orbital-ethmoid fractures. JAMA Facial Plast Surg 2014;16(4):284–9.
6. Strong EB, Buchalter GM, Moulthrop THM. Endoscopic repair of isolated anterior table frontal sinus fractures. Arch Facial Plast Surg 2003;5(6):514–21.

7. Strong EB, Shaye DA, Steele TO, et al. Frontal sinus fractures: a surgical management paradigm. Oto-rino-laringologia (Bucuresti 1990) 2017;67(1):10–25.
8. Strong EB. Frontal sinus fractures: current concepts. Craniomaxillofacial Trauma Reconstr 2009;2(3–4):161–75.
9. Smith TL, Han JK, Loehrl TA, et al. Endoscopic management of the frontal recess in frontal sinus fractures: a shift in the paradigm? Laryngoscope 2002;112(5): 784–90.
10. Grayson JW, Jeyarajan H, Illing EA, et al. Changing the surgical dogma in frontal sinus trauma: transnasal endoscopic repair: endoscopic repair of frontal sinus trauma. Int Forum Allergy Rhinol 2017;7(5):441–9.
11. Langlie J, Kim M, Thaller SR. Frontal sinus fractures: a review on etiology and management emphasizing minimally invasive and endoscopic techniques. J Craniofac Surg 2021;32(3):1246–50.
12. Choi KJ, Chang B, Woodard CR, et al. Survey of current practice patterns in the management of frontal sinus fractures. Craniomaxillofacial Trauma Reconstr 2017;10(2):106–16.
13. Le P, Martinez R, Black J. Frontal sinus fracture management meta-analysis: endoscopic versus open repair. J Craniofac Surg 2021;32(4):1311–5.
14. Villwock JA, Suryadevara AC. Update on approaches to the craniomaxillofacial skeleton. Curr Opin Otolaryngol Head Neck Surg 2014;22(4):326–31.
15. Ha YI, Kim SH, Park ES, et al. Approach for naso-orbito-ethmoidal fracture. Arch Craniofacial Surg 2019;20(4):219–22.
16. Vujcich N, Gebauer D. Current and evolving trends in the management of facial fractures. Aust Dent J 2018;63:S35–47.
17. Kakizaki H, Takahashi Y, Miyazaki H, et al. Swinging eyelid procedure: an useful approach for reduction of zygomaticomalar fracture. Surg Sci 2011;02(03):147–50.
18. De Riu G, Meloni SM, Gobbi R, et al. Subciliary versus swinging eyelid approach to the orbital floor. J Cranio-Maxillo-Fac Surg 2008;36(8):439–42.
19. Homer N, Huggins A, Durairaj VD. Contemporary management of orbital blowout fractures. Curr Opin Otolaryngol Head Neck Surg 2019;27(4):310–6.
20. Rhee JS, Lynch J, Loehrl TA. Intranasal endoscopy-assisted repair of medial orbital wall fractures. Arch Facial Plast Surg 2000;2(4):269–73.
21. Rhee JS, Chen CT. Endoscopic approach to medial orbital wall fractures. Facial Plast Surg Clin North Am 2006;14(1):17–23.
22. Bonsembiante A, Valente L, Ciorba A, et al. Transnasal endoscopic approach for the treatment of medial orbital wall fractures. Ann Maxillofac Surg 2019;9(2):411.
23. Farwell DG, Strong EB. Endoscopic repair of orbital floor fractures. Otolaryngol Clin North Am 2007;40(2):319–28.
24. Cheong EC, Chen CT, Chen YR. Broad application of the endoscope for orbital floor reconstruction: long-term follow-up results. Plast Reconstr Surg 2010; 125(3):969–78.
25. Balakrishnan K, Moe KS. Applications and outcomes of orbital and transorbital endoscopic surgery. Otolaryngol Neck Surg 2011;144(5):815–20.
26. Nastri AL, Gurney B. Current concepts in midface fracture management. Curr Opin Otolaryngol Head Neck Surg 2016;24(4):368–75.
27. Louis M, Agrawal N, Kaufman M, et al. Midface fractures I. Semin Plast Surg 2017;31(02):085–93.
28. Peretti N, MacLeod S. Zygomaticomaxillary complex fractures: diagnosis and treatment. Curr Opin Otolaryngol Head Neck Surg 2017;25(4):314–9.
29. Weiss JP, Sawhney R. Update on mandibular condylar fracture management. Curr Opin Otolaryngol Head Neck Surg 2016;24(4):273–8.

30. Landa L, Tartan B, Acartuk A, et al. The transcervical incision for use in oral and maxillofacial surgical procedures. J Oral Maxillofac Surg 2003;61(3):343–6.

31. Wilson A, Ethunandan M, Brennan P. Transmasseteric antero-parotid approach for open reduction and internal fixation of condylar fractures. Br J Oral Maxillofac Surg 2005;43(1):57–60.

32. Narayanan V, Ramadorai A, Ravi P, et al. Transmasseteric anterior parotid approach for condylar fractures. Br J Oral Maxillofac Surg 2012;50(5):420–4.

33. Ducic Y. Endoscopic treatment of subcondylar fractures. Laryngoscope 2008; 118(7):1164–7.

Nasal Fractures: Acute, Subacute, and Delayed Management

Oscar Trujillo, MD, MS[a],*, Clara Lee, MD[a]

KEYWORDS

- Nasal fracture • Closed reduction • Delayed treatment • Septal fracture

KEY POINTS

- Nasal fractures compose nearly 50% of all facial fractures and can vary in pattern based on the direction of impact.
- Although x-rays are more cost-effective, computed tomography scan remains the gold standard diagnostic tool, particularly if other facial fractures are suspected.
- Closed reduction of nasal fractures in an acute setting may be a useful first-line treatment, but subsequent/secondary interventions have been reported in the literature in 11% to 50% of cases.
- Open reduction in a delayed fashion may be more useful for complex or open nasal fractures, fractures with significant dorsal or caudal septum involvement, and fractures involving the internal nasal valve.
- Treatment of nasal fractures can vary greatly based on the timing of presentation, degree or nature of the fracture, patient goals, and surgeon experience.

INTRODUCTION

The nose plays a critical role in facial appearance and respiratory function. Its prominent location places the nose at risk for injuries from various mechanisms, including sports-related injuries, motor vehicle accidents, and assaults. Nasal fractures account for nearly 50% of all facial fractures, with the greatest incidence in young males.[1] Nasal fractures occur in several distinct patterns based on the direction of the impact. Anterior forces can result in widening of the nasal bones, whereas laterally directed forces can result in C- or S-shaped deformities. Nasal fractures can occur in isolation or in conjunction with other facial fractures, including frontal, midface, or naso-orbitoethmoid fractures. In this article, the authors review the management of nasal fractures.

[a] Department of Otolaryngology–Head & Neck Surgery, Columbia University Irving Medical Center, 180 Fort Washington Avenue HP8, New York, NY 10032, USA
* Corresponding author.
E-mail address: ot2166@cumc.columbia.edu

Otolaryngol Clin N Am 56 (2023) 1089–1099
https://doi.org/10.1016/j.otc.2023.05.004
0030-6665/23/Published by Elsevier Inc.

oto.theclinics.com

ANATOMY

A detailed understanding of nasal anatomy is critical to the assessment and treatment of nasal fractures. The nose can be divided into thirds: the upper bony vault, middle cartilaginous vault, and nasal tip. The upper bony vault is composed of paired nasal bones, which contact the frontal bone superiorly at the nasion. The deepest point of the nasal bone is the radix (or sellion). Caudally, the nasal bones contact the paired upper lateral cartilages at the rhinion, which is referred to as the "keystone area." Together, the nasal bones and upper lateral cartilages provide shape and structure to the nasal dorsum. In the middle vault, the upper lateral cartilages attach to the septum at the midline, providing support for the internal nasal valve. The upper lateral cartilages articulate with the lower lateral cartilages at the scroll region, which serves as a major tip support mechanism. In the lower third of the nose, the paired lower lateral cartilages define the nasal tip and support the external nasal valve, as shown in **Fig. 1.**[2]

The left and right nasal cavities are divided by the nasal septum. The septum is built of quadrangular cartilage anteriorly, vomer posteroinferiorly, and perpendicular plate of the ethmoid posterosuperiorly, as shown in **Fig. 2.**[3] Inferiorly, the nasal septum attaches to the nasal spine and maxillary crest with thick decussating fibers, which provide support and stability. The nasal septum develops until age 12 to 13 years; therefore, injury to the nasal septum during childhood may result in midface growth abnormalities. The septum houses ample vascular supply, which can lead to significant epistaxis with nasal trauma. In the anterior septum, the Kiesselbach plexus is formed from contributions from the anterior and posterior ethmoid arteries, sphenopalatine artery, greater palatine artery, and superior labial artery. In the posterior septum, the Woodruff plexus is formed from anastomoses of the sphenopalatine and ascending pharyngeal arteries. Sensation to the nose is provided by branches of the trigeminal nerve. The ophthalmic branch (V1) provides sensation to the nasal dorsum and tip. The maxillary nerve provides sensation to the ala and columella (V2).

EVALUATION

The examination of a trauma patient always begins with airway, breathing, and circulation. Once the patient has been stabilized, a focused examination for nasal trauma can be performed. Relevant aspects of the history include the mechanism and timing

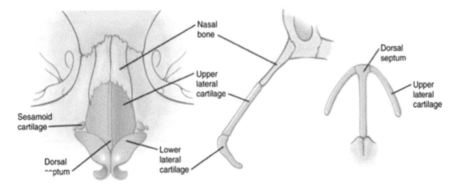

Fig. 1. Nasal anatomy showing upper, middle, and lower thirds. (McCarn KE, Downs BW, Cook TA, et al. The middle vault: upper lateral cartilage modifications. In: Azizzadeh B, Murphy MR, Johnson CM, et al, editors. Master techniques in rhinoplasty. Philadelphia: Saunders; 2011. p. 159-67).

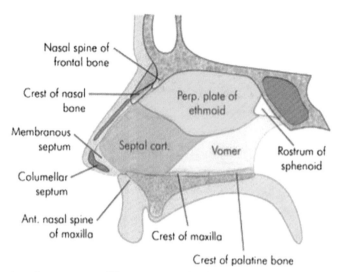

Fig. 2. Nasal septum anatomy. (Sharma AR et al. Clinical outcome following septoplasty with or without turbinate reduction. *Int J Otorhinolargyngol Head Neck Surg.* 2020;6(9):1651-1658.)

of injury as well as the presence of nasal obstruction, clear rhinorrhea, epistaxis, or visual changes. Inquiring about any prior nasal injuries, nasal surgery, preexisting nasal obstruction, or deformity may be useful as well. The nasal skin should be examined for any edema, ecchymosis, crepitus, or lacerations. Significant soft tissue swelling may obscure accurate examination of the nasal framework. The upper third of the nose should be examined for collapse, deviation, or widening of the nasal bones. Discontinuity of the upper lateral cartilages from the nasal bones may result in an "inverted V" deformity. Injury to the caudal septum may cause displacement off the maxillary crest and associated nasal tip deviation.

Anterior rhinoscopy and nasal endoscopy should also be performed. The use of vasoconstricting agents, such as oxymetazoline, may be helpful if there is concurrent epistaxis. The nasal septum should be examined for any mucosal tears, septal fractures, or hematoma. In particular, the timely identification of septal hematomas is critical for preventing superinfection, cartilage necrosis, and resultant "saddle nose" deformity.

If there is a hematoma, it must quickly be evacuated and nasal packing placed to prevent re-accumulation of fluid. If the cartilage of the septum is separated from the perichondrium where it receives its blood supply by fluid or a hematoma, it will undergo necrosis or become an abscess resulting in a septal defect, loss of dorsal height, or saddle nose deformity. Although rare, consistent clear rhinorrhea should raise suspicion for cerebrospinal fluid leak and skull base injury. Formal endoscopic evaluation may be difficult in the acute setting due to edema and bleeding.

Finally, the remainder of the facial bones should be carefully examined for signs of additional fractures, including naso-orbitoethmoid, midface, or frontal bone fractures. Radiographic imaging is generally not indicated in isolated nasal bone fractures. On occasion, emergency rooms may perform nasal x-rays with Waters view or lateral nasal views as quick diagnostic tests (which is more cost-efficient than a computed tomography [CT] scan) if an isolated nasal fracture is suspected. **Fig. 3**A and B shows a Waters view and lateral nasal view, respectively, of the nasal bones with a fracture.

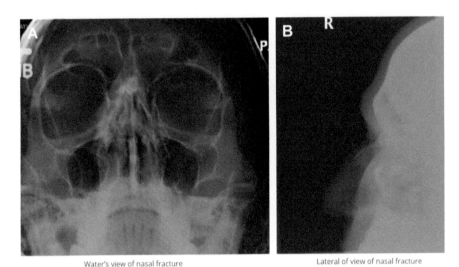

Water's view of nasal fracture   Lateral of view of nasal fracture

Fig. 3. Nasal x-ray showing an acute nasal fracture in Waters (*A*) and lateral views (*B*).

However, in cases of diagnostic uncertainty or suspicion for multiple facial fractures, CT maxillofacial scans may be useful.

In a 6-year study looking at over 500 nasal fractures, nasal x-rays were reliable at diagnosing nasal fractures in 82% of the cases and were falsely negative compared with CT scans in 9.5% of their cases.[4] Also in this study, the investigators observed distinct nasal fracture patterns seen on CT scan with the most common pattern being a unilateral displaced nasal fracture without septal involvement (36%) followed by bilateral displaced fractures involving the septum (21%). The patterns of fracture on CT can be seen in **Fig. 4**.[4] Interesting, the false negatives on nasal x-ray were noted as type IIA fracture patterns on CT 50% of the time in their study. Although in this study x-rays were able to pick up many nasal fractures, the gold standard for diagnosing nasal fractures is by CT and it is also reported that around half of nasal fractures are associated with other facial fractures for which a CT would be more helpful to diagnose.[5] When reviewing CT scans for nasal fractures, the axial view on bone window is the most optimal to evaluate nasal bone depression, displacement, deviation, comminution, and septal involvement.

MANAGEMENT
Acute Nasal Fractures

In the management of nasal fractures, the need for intervention is determined by the degree of nasal obstruction and nasal deformity. Also, in considering management, it is reported that around two-thirds of nasal fractures involve the frontal process of the maxilla and 42% have associated septal fractures.[5] Therefore, the surgeon must consider the effect of fractures on these areas. The surgeon must determine the best treatment (observation versus closed or open reduction), timing of intervention, and appropriate anesthetic (local versus general).

As a first line, patients experiencing new-onset mild nasal obstruction or nasal deformity should be offered a closed reduction. Closed reduction is a conservative measure that may improve aesthetic outcomes and decrease the extent of septal deviation.[6,7] Closed reduction is indicated if there is a visible deformity following the injury and is particularly useful if there is significant deviation or depression of the nasal

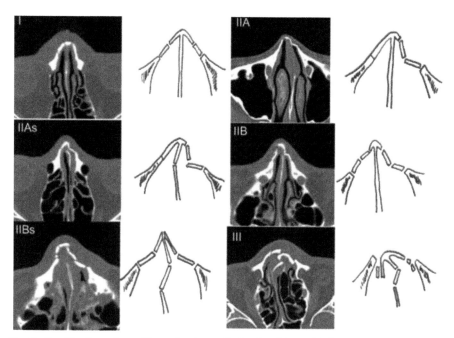

Fig. 4. Classification of nasal bone fractures: (I) simple without displacement (8%); (IIA) simple with displacement/without telescoping unilateral (36%); (IIAs) unilateral with septal fracture (13%); (IIB) bilateral (18%); (IIBs) bilateral with septal fracture (21%); (III) comminuted with telescoping or depression (4%). (Hwang K et al. Analysis of nasal bone fractures; A six-year study of 503 patients. Journal of Craniofacial Surgery. 2006; 17 (2):2161-264.)

bones. Before performing a closed reduction, the surgeon must review the CT scan to rule out a concomitant fracture at the cribriform plate to reduce the risk of causing a cerebrospinal fluid (CSF) leak or olfactory cleft damage.[5]

When performing a closed reduction, it is important to weigh the options of the use of local anesthetic or general anesthetic to perform the procedure. Local anesthetic has the obvious advantage of reducing the overall risks associated with general anesthesia as well as the ease of timing of the procedure if it can be done bedside or in the office. However, even with trigeminal nerve blocks, anxiolytics, oral pain management, and intranasal topical anesthetics, the surgeon cannot be as aggressive with manipulation of the nasal bones without causing the patient discomfort under local anesthetic. A meta-analysis study performed on comparison of the two modalities of anesthetic for closed reductions of nasal fractures found that although the overall cost of general anesthetic is higher, patient satisfaction in aesthetic and functional outcome was higher with this modality.[8] Also, patients who underwent reduction with general anesthetic were less likely to require secondary procedures/corrections.[8] Therefore, closed reduction under local anesthetic should be reserved for patients in which the deformity can be reasonably corrected, the patient can tolerate the procedure either bedside or in the office, or if the patient cannot receive general anesthetic for other medical reasons.

In a large population-based study, the rate of septorhinoplasty after closed reduction was 1.6%; however, a different study found that as many as 29% of patients reported initial dissatisfaction with aesthetic outcomes after closed reduction and said they would consider further surgery. In other studies, the need for secondary septorhinoplasty after closed reduction was reported in 11% to 50% of patients.[9] Careful patient selection may help maximize a surgeon's chances of performing a successful closed reduction. Patient factors, such as preexisting nasal obstruction and the presence of a septal fracture, have been shown to increase the likelihood of persistent nasal obstruction and need for future septorhinoplasty.[10–12] It is important to counsel patients that they may ultimately need further surgery to achieve optimal results if they opt to do a closed reduction under local anesthetic. Photo documentation is critical in these situations.

The ideal timing for a closed reduction occurs after nasal soft tissue swelling has subsided, but before the nasal bones have healed. If a significant soft tissue swelling is present, it may be difficult to accurately evaluate the patient's anatomy and perform an appropriate reduction. In the immediate setting, a closed reduction may be possible if the patient seeks care within 3 to 6 hours of the injury, before swelling sets in. Beyond this timeframe, it is generally recommended to delay reduction until swelling resolves, for up to 14 days in adults (7 days typically in the pediatric population). However, recent literature suggests that some improvement may still be achieved with a closed reduction performed up to 5 weeks after initial injury.[13]

Closed reductions are performed in various settings depending on the practice and surgeon preference, including bedside in an inpatient setting or in the office. The most common instrument used is a Boies elevator placed intranasally between the septum and nasal bone to mobilize the nasal bones back into position. Where there is no elevator available, manual pressure can be used within the 14-day window to mobilize the relatively mobile nasal bones, especially if their septum cartilage is not significantly deviated. Where there is a concomitant septal cartilage deviation, Walsham or Asch forceps are generally used as they allow for controlled stabilization and mobilization of the septum itself on both sides to correct the deviation back onto the maxillary crest in the midline.[5]

After mobilization of the septum cartilage, some form of splinting or fixation intranasally must be placed (either Doyle silicone splints or Merocel nonabsorbable packing) for 5 to 7 days to allow the septum to heal in its new position. Nasal endoscopy both before and after manipulation should be used to confirm that the deviated septum has been corrected. An external cast should also be placed to help avoid further trauma to the area and to simply remind patients to take care with their nose after manipulation.

Subacute or Delayed Fractures

Patients who have suffered nasal fractures but have not had intervention in the first 10 to 14 days, but are less than 3 months since their fracture, fall into the subacute fracture category. There can be a variety of reasons why patients did not or could not seek intervention in the acute phase and subacute or chronic/delay fractures commonly present in clinic or outpatient settings. Some literature advocates that if patients are not treated in the acute phase (10–14 days) they wait at least 6 weeks before surgical intervention to allow for all the swelling and inflammation from the fracture to subside.[9] These may also be patients with unresolved nasal or septal deformities after closed reductions. Studies find that the most common cause of secondary interventions after a closed reduction is an unreduced septal fracture.[9]

In cases of severe injury, closed reduction may be inadequate, and an open approach is required. The examples of such scenarios include extensive fracturing of the nasal bones, open septal fractures, nasal valve collapse, severe dislocation of the caudal or dorsal septum, or prior failed closed reduction. Fundamentally, a surgeon must consider whether the septum can be adequately reduced back onto the nasal/maxillary crest with a closed reduction or if the involvement of the maxillary spine has destabilized the caudal septum off the midline, in which case an open approach combined with septoplasty is more appropriate. In a retrospective review of 49 patients with both nasal bone and septal fractures, the investigators showed a lower revision rate (75% vs 6.5%) in open approaches to the bony pyramid combined with septoplasty compared with closed reduction alone.[14] Some also advocate that if there is a septal injury or deviation of the nasal bridge greater than 50%, a closed reduction is not sufficient and septoplasty must be performed concomitantly with open reduction of the nasal bones.[14]

To illustrate, **Fig. 5**A and B shows a patient of the senior author who presented with a nasal and septal fracture with significant dorsal septal deviation of more than 50%, internal nasal valve collapse, and significant nasal bony deviation requiring a delayed treatment with open septorhinoplasty, internal nasal valve repair with spreader grafts, and open reduction of nasal bones before and 3 months after repair.

Where a fracture results in damage to the key portions of the septal L-strut (such as the dorsal or caudal 1 cm strip) or deviation of the cartilaginous nasal bridge, the best course of treatment is a delayed open septorhinoplasty approach.[14] Such septal injuries can result in a significant deviation of the external appearance of the nose in the cartilaginous portion, and those areas are especially important for maintaining nasal support and nasal tip support. **Fig. 6**A and B shows a patient of the senior author with a significant caudal septal fracture that required an open septorhinoplasty/reconstruction and who was not an appropriate candidate for a closed reduction alone. As such, the patient's treatment was delayed for 3 months until his nose could heal from the fracture to permit reconstruction sufficient to improve his breathing and reestablish support to his nasal tip. Delayed open septorhinoplasty is also preferred where there is internal nasal valve collapse, which can be determined on a positive Cottle maneuver on examination after the injury. This typically occurs when there is a fracture at the

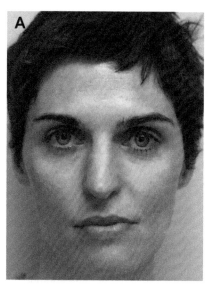 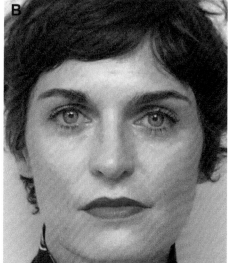

Preoperative nasal/septal fracture   3 months post operative

Fig. 5. Patient of the senior author before and after delayed treatment of nasal bone and dorsal septal L-strut fracture.

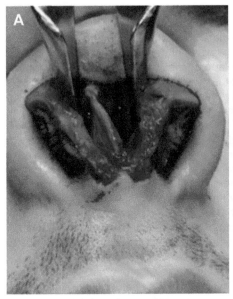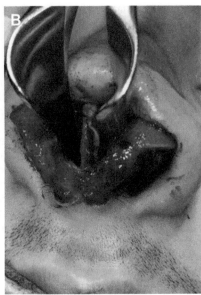

Pre Reconstruction   Immediately Post Reconstruction

Fig. 6. Patient of the senior author before and immediately after delayed repair of caudal septal L-strut fracture.

junction between the upper lateral cartilage and nasal bone. If there is internal nasal valve collapse, a closed reduction will not address this issue.

Septorhinoplasty is generally delayed 3 to 6 months following fracture to allow adequate time for the nasal bones and cartilages to rest in their final positions and to allow any skin or septal mucosal lacerations to heal. The literature also supports that an open approach is better suited to address nasal fractures accompanied by even more complex facial fractures, such as naso-orbito-ethmoid (NOE) or Le Fort II/III fractures. There is, however, some dispute as to whether isolated nasal fractures should be treated closed before open treatment. Currently, the literature accepts the indication of delayed open treatment of nasal bones (or more precisely, open septo-rhinoplasty for nasal/septal fractures) for severe septal cartilaginous fractures, comminuted nasal bone fractures, severe nasal bone fractures (eg, implicating the NOE or LeFort), or those that destabilize the nasal framework (eg, dorsal or caudal septal fractures).

There is also some discord as to the timing of intervention. The proponents of early intervention with closed reductions in the acute phase argue that it helps to achieve early skeletal stabilization/correction, prevents late nasal deformities and osseous malunion, and mitigates against soft tissue scarring/contracture that can complicate a delayed treatment course. On the other hand, the proponents of delayed open treatment urge that the delay permits the fracture to fully heal, resulting in increased septal cartilage to use for grafting, reduced inflammation, and the healing of mucosal lacerations. As such, the surgeon is able to more rigidly fix and/or reduce the fracture in a controlled way with improved visualization.

Table 1 provides the general guidelines suggesting timing of intervention and intervention approaches described in the literature based on the nature and timing of

Table 1
Management of isolated nasal fractures

Nasal Fracture Presentation	Bony Deformity Without Septal Involvement	Bony Deformity + Mild Septal Involvement	Bony Deformity + Caudal or Dorsal L-Strut Septal Involvement	Bony Deformity + Nasal Valve Collapse (+Cottle Maneuver)	Complex Bony Deformity + Open External Lacerations
Acute (<2 wk)	Closed reduction	Can consider closed reduction as first-line treatment	Delay treatment	Delay treatment	Delay treatment
Subacute (6 wk–3 mo)	Open reduction	Open reduction +/- septoplasty if airway obstruction present	Delay treatment	Delay treatment	Delay treatment
Chronic/Delayed (>3 mo)	Open reduction	Open reduction +/- septoplasty if airway obstruction present	Open septorhinoplasty with open reduction	Open septorhinoplasty repair of nasal valve with open reduction	Open septorhinoplasty with open reduction

fracture presentation. The guidelines below, however, do not consider how treatment decisions may also be affected by patient goals and preference or experience of the treating surgeon. Nonetheless, the below provides a framework for evaluating isolated nasal fractures and may be helpful in patient counseling regarding treatment options.

Pediatric Nasal Fractures

Pediatric nasal fractures (<12 years old) merit different consideration regarding timing and treatment than adult nasal fractures. Although pediatric nasal fractures are the most common facial fracture in the pediatric population, they are not very common in general. This is due to their underdeveloped facial skeleton, thick overlying soft tissue, and general close supervision by their parents.[15]

The current consensus is that pediatric nasal fractures generally need earlier intervention than adults in the range of 3 to 7 days after the initial trauma, given their fast-healing rate and osteogenesis of their facial skeleton. Pediatric nasal fractures are more difficult to detect with x-ray because they have underdeveloped nasal bones and thick overlying soft tissue. CT is a better modality but exposes children to higher levels of ionizing radiation, which is to be discouraged.

In a recent study evaluating 98 pediatric patients that either underwent early intervention (3–7 days) or delayed intervention (>7 days), they found no significant difference in patient outcomes.[15] Outcomes were determined by postoperative CT evaluation of nasal bone alignment and nasal bone deformities post-intervention. All patients included were 12 years old or younger, and all received closed reductions under general anesthesia. Those excluded were pediatric patients who had previous nasal fractures, previous nasal surgery, or a nasal fracture concomitant with other facial fractures at the time of presentation. Forty-two of the fifty-one patients (82.4%) who had early treatment (3–7 days) showed excellent outcomes, defined as no bony malalignment of the fracture segment or bony irregularities.[15] Thirty-nine of the forty-seven patients (83%) in the delayed treatment group (<7 days) showed excellent outcomes.[15] Patients without septal injury were significantly more likely to have excellent outcomes. In the delayed treatment group, almost all were performed within 2 weeks except for two cases performed at 18 and 25 days after injury. Also importantly in their study, no septal manipulation or septoplasty was performed for fear of disrupting the growth centers in the nose. Only bony manipulation or reduction was performed under general anesthesia. The authors of this study even advocate that for a child who is 2 to 3 weeks post-isolated nasal fracture, there may still be some advantage to attempting a closed reduction of the nasal bones under general anesthesia.

SUMMARY

Nasal fractures are very common. Treatment timing and technique varies from patient-to-patient and surgeon-to-surgeon. The literature describes early intervention (<14 days) with closed techniques as cost-effective, minimizing the need for possible secondary surgeries and improved early patient satisfaction. However, the authors observe a measurably high rate of subsequent open treatment after closed treatment, particularly where there is significant septal involvement in the fracture. Moreover, delayed intervention (>3 months) with an open approach has many advantages over early closed technique, including a lower revision rate, improved ability for rigid fixation and support, and the ability to correct severe dorsal or caudal L-strut deformities, nasal valve issues, and severe nasal bony deviation/deformities. These observations should inform the discussion of treatment options between the surgeon and the patient to ensure the best possible surgical outcome.

DISCLOUSRE

The authors have nothing to disclose.

REFERENCES

1. Basheeth N, Donnelly M, David S, et al. Acute nasal fracture management: a prospective study and literature review. Laryngoscope 2015;125(12):2677–84.
2. Hsu DW, Suh JD. Anatomy and physiology of nasal obstruction. Otolaryngol Clin North Am 2018;51:853–65.
3. Sharma AR, Jain S, Sen K, et al. Clinical outcome following septoplasty with or without turbinate reduction. Int J Otorhinolargyngol Head Neck Surg 2020;6(9): 1651–8.
4. Hwang K, You SH, Kim SG, et al. Analysis of nasal bone fractures; a six-year study of 503 patients. J Craniofac Surg 2006;17(2):261–4.
5. Landeen KC, Kimura K, Stephan SJ. Nasal fractures. Facial Plast Surg Clin N AM 2022;30:23–30.
6. Plath M, Cavaliere C, Seide S, et al. Does a closed reduction improve aesthetical and functional outcome after nasal fracture? Eur Arch Oto-Rhino-Laryngol 2023; 280(5):2299–308.
7. Choi JH, Oh HM, Hwang JH, et al. Do closed reduction and fracture patterns of the nasal bone affect nasal septum deviation? Arch Craniofac Surg 2022;23(3): 119–24.
8. Al-Moraissi EA, Ellis E 3rd. Local versus general anesthesia for the management of nasal bone fractures: a systematic review and meta-analysis. J Oral Maxillofac Surg 2015;73(4):606–15.
9. Davis RE, Chu E. Complex nasal fractures in the Adult-A changing management philosophy. Facial Plast Surg 2015;31(3):201–15.
10. Hung T, Chang W, Vlantis AC, et al. Patient satisfaction after closed reduction of nasal fractures. Arch Facial Plast Surg 2007;9(1):40–3.
11. Li K, Moubayed SP, Spataro E, et al. Risk factors for corrective septorhinoplasty associated with initial treatment of isolated nasal fracture. JAMA Facial Plast Surg 2018;20(6):460–7.
12. Arnold MA, Yanik SC, Suryadevara AC. Septal fractures predict poor outcomes after closed nasal reduction: retrospective review and survey. Laryngoscope 2019;129(8):1784–90.
13. Yoon HY, Han DG. Delayed reduction of nasal bone fractures. Arch Craniofac Surg 2016;17(2):51–5.
14. Lu GN, Humphrey CD, Kriet JD. Correction of nasal fractures. Facial Plast Surg Clin N AM 2017;25:537–46.
15. Kang WK, Han DG, Kim S-E, et al. Comparison of postoperative outcomes between early and delayed surgery for pediatric nasal fractures. Arch Craniofac Surg 2021;22(2):93–8.

Current Guidelines and Opinions in the Management of Orbital Floor Fractures

Radha P. Pandya, BS[a], Wenyu Deng, MD[a,b],
Nickisa M. Hodgson, MD[a,b],*

KEYWORDS

- Orbital floor fracture • Transconjunctival • Subciliary • Orbital implants • Titanium
- Porous polyethylene

KEY POINTS

- Orbital floor fractures commonly result from facial trauma and can either be isolated or involve multiple sites.
- Surgical intervention should be determined based on absolute indications for repair, including tissue entrapment, persistent diplopia, clinically significant enophthalmos, and large fractures.
- In the absence of indications for immediate repair, surgical intervention should be delayed to at least 1 to 2 weeks after injury to allow for resolution of edema but performed before advancement of scarring and fibrosis.
- When surgical repair is indicated, the transconjunctival approach is most widely favored due to better outcomes and less scarring and complications.
- Implant materials vary and are often dependent on surgeon training and preference.

INTRODUCTION

Orbital floor fractures are a painful and disabling result of blunt trauma to the face, commonly causing emergency department visits. Orbital and periorbital trauma accounts for approximately 3% of emergency department visits, which are commonly the result of assault, motor vehicle accidents, sports, and falls.[1] Of patients with facial fractures with computed tomography (CT), 49% were found to have an orbital fracture.

---

[a] Department of Ophthalmology, SUNY Downstate Medical Center, 450 Clarkson Avenue, Brooklyn, NY 11203, USA; [b] Department of Ophthalmology, Kings County Medical Center, 451 Clarkson Avenue, Brooklyn, NY 11203, USA
* Corresponding author. Department of Ophthalmology, SUNY Downstate Medical Center, 450 Clarkson Avenue, MSC 58, Brooklyn, NY 11203.
E-mail address: nickisa.hodgson@downstate.edu

Otolaryngol Clin N Am 56 (2023) 1101–1112
https://doi.org/10.1016/j.otc.2023.05.002
0030-6665/23/© 2023 Elsevier Inc. All rights reserved.

Orbital fractures were commonly found in conjunction with other facial fractures and were frequently found to involve multiple fractures of the orbital walls. The orbital floor was the most common fracture site, composing 47.9% of all orbital fractures, followed by medial wall, lateral wall, and roof fractures. Young adults were most frequently affected, with the prevalence decreasing with each subsequent decade of life.[1] A second retrospective study found similar epidemiologic results, with patients between 15 and 35 years making up 37.5% of the patient collective.[2]

Orbital fractures can occur in isolation or involve multiple sites, including orbital floor, medial wall, lateral wall, and roof. The orbit is composed of seven bones (**Fig. 1**). The orbital roof is formed from the frontal and sphenoid bones, the medial wall is formed from the lacrimal, ethmoid, maxillary, and sphenoid bones, and the lateral wall comprises the sphenoid and zygomatic bones and considered the strongest wall. Finally, the orbital floor is composed of the maxillary, palatine, and zygomatic bones.[3] There have been several proposed fracture classification systems, including a system identified by Hammer in 1995 that describes orbital fractures with the development of other facial fractures. In this system, Type I fractures (orbito-zygomatic fractures) involve orbital walls and the zygomatic complex, Type II fractures (internal orbital fractures) include isolated orbital fractures, Type III fractures (naso-orbito-ethmoid-type fractures) involve the naso-orbital-ethmoid complex, and Type IV fractures (complex fractures) include more extensive panfacial fractures.[4] Other systems classify fractures based on energy of impact, degree of displacement of structures, and involvement of the orbital rims.[5] Although this review only discusses orbital floor fractures, it is important to recognize the complexity of the orbit and associated fracture patterns.

Currently, there are two prevailing theories outlining the biomechanics of injury in orbital floor fractures. The first is the retropulsion theory, proposed in 1944, which suggests that blunt impact causes a sudden rise in the intraorbital pressure transmitting

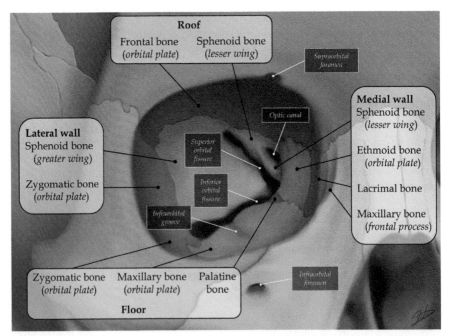

Fig. 1. Key landmarks and anatomic details of the orbit. (Illustrated by Wenyu Deng, MD.)

forces along the orbital walls, ultimately resulting in fractures in the areas of the least thickness.[6] The second is the buckling theory, which states that sudden blunt impact causes a ripple of forces through the orbital floor, causing a compression in the anteroposterior direction and a fracture commonly in the posteromedial aspect of the orbital floor.[7] Both theories identify the orbital floor as the weakest region of the orbit and thus most prone to injury.

Management of orbital fractures, including indications for surgery, remains a controversial topic. Extraocular muscle and orbital tissue entrapment are a clear indication for urgent surgical repair (**Fig. 2**). Further, there are three commonly agreed on guidelines for surgical repair: (1) persistent diplopia in primary or reading position, (2) clinically significant enophthalmos greater than 2 mm, and (3) fracture involving greater than 50% of the orbital floor.[8] However, debate remains regarding exact indications for repair, timing of intervention, the role of intraoperative and postoperative imaging, and preferred implant type. In addition, the interdisciplinary nature of orbital fractures requires multiple specialties to be familiar with its management, including ophthalmology, facial plastics, and otolaryngology.

This article reviews the current guidelines for orbital floor fracture repair among multiple specialties. Specifically, the authors discuss current indications for surgical repair, timing of intervention, outpatient versus inpatient management, the role of intraoperative and postoperative imaging, and choice of implant material.

INDICATIONS FOR REPAIR

There has been significant discussion regarding indications for surgical reconstruction. A recent review defined absolute indications of intervention as (1) immediate clinical enophthalmos due to poorer outcomes from progressive atrophy of intra-orbital fat, (2) severe restriction in ocular motility due to muscle entrapment or soft tissue incarceration, and (3) "white-eye blowout" fracture in a pediatric patient (ie, orbital fracture with tissue entrapment in the fracture, causing restrictive strabismus) and vagal symptoms. Relative indications for repair were defined as (1) defects involving at least 50% of the orbital floor or a 20 × 20 mm size of the defect and/or (2) non-resolving and persistent diplopia for at least 2 weeks due to soft tissue entrapment or fibrosis.[5] Similarly, a second review included diplopia for 2 weeks and a fracture involving more than half of the orbital floor as absolute indications along with enophthalmos for 2 weeks.[8] Parameswaran and colleagues[5] also specified relative contraindications for surgical repair, including (1) associated ophthalmic injuries (eg, retinal tears, hyphema, displacement of the lens, ruptured globe, and avulsion injuries of the globe) and (2) loss of vision in the non-fractured eye. Other studies have simply

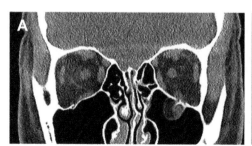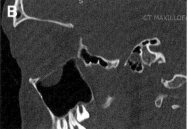

Fig. 2. Coronal (*A*) and sagittal (*B*) computed tomography (CT) scan demonstrating left orbital floor fracture with entrapment of the inferior rectus.

stated that indications for surgery are based on clinical examination findings, orbital imaging, and assessment of the risks and benefits.[9] In a recent survey by Aldekhayel and colleagues, six factors were found to have the greatest influence on a surgeon's operative decision—enophthalmos, hypophthalmos, positive forced duction, defect size, motility restriction, and persistent diplopia. In addition, one-third of participants reported being less likely to operate on orbital floor fractures now versus earlier in their careers, indicating improved guidelines and more conservative approaches.[10]

Basta and colleagues proposed a risk stratification tool for predicting the need for surgical intervention. Their study demonstrated that orbital volume change is more predictive of need for surgical intervention than the size of the fracture defect. In addition, they suggest that inferior rectus displacement at or inferior to the fracture line can serve as a predictive marker (**Fig. 3**). These predictors likely improve the detection of clinically significant enophthalmos and persistent diplopia and should be considered in the evaluation of patients with orbital floor fractures.[11]

Among the different specialties, indications for repair are similar. In a survey of oculoplastics and facial plastics, the most important surgical indications for both were found to be motility restriction, enophthalmos, and diplopia at 2 weeks. Facial plastic surgeons placed emphasis on enophthalmos, considering this a "very strong factor" in their decision to operate, whereas oculoplastic surgeons considered it "moderately or strongly" influential.[12] Similarly, the greatest influencing indicators for surgery among oral and maxillofacial surgeons were defect size greater than 2 cm^2, enophthalmos, muscle or soft tissue entrapment, and persistent diplopia.[13]

TIMING OF INTERVENTION

The timing of surgical intervention can be more complex, namely in allowing enough time for the resolution of swelling of the infraorbital and periorbital tissues while intervening early enough to reduce postoperative complications. This balance rests on the idea that deferring surgery to reduce periorbital edema mitigates the risk of compartment syndrome and allows for improvement in clinical symptoms but also increases the risk of fibrosis and chronic diplopia.[9] General recommendations state best practice is to allow 1 to 2 weeks for observation in case of spontaneous resolution of edema and the presenting symptoms, and then performing the surgery as close to 2 weeks from the trauma date as possible to allow for further reduction in swelling and easier exploration of the orbit before scarring and fibrosis advances. However,

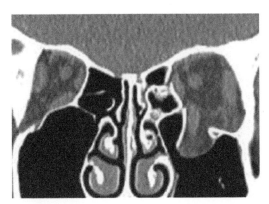

Fig. 3. Coronal CT scan demonstrating large left orbital floor fracture with herniation of orbital contents.

the 2 week rule is debated with many surgeons advocating similar outcomes with later intervention.[2,8,14]

Intervention can be broken down into immediate intervention and delayed intervention within approximately 14 days. According to Seifert and colleagues,[2] indications for immediate intervention are early enophthalmos with facial asymmetry and signs of the oculocardiac reflex, or decreased vision in the affected eye. Although early enophthalmos and oculocardiac reflex are clear indications for early surgery, decreased visual acuity in the early post-trauma period can be due to a multitude of reasons, including but not limited to traumatic optic neuropathy, commotio retinae, periorbital edema, retrobulbar hemorrhage (RBH), and should not be an indication for fracture repair. Boyette and colleagues provided the following guidelines for immediate repair: (1) presence of the oculocardiac reflex, (2) muscle entrapment, and (3) significant enophthalmos at the time of the injury. The oculocardiac reflex is a reduction in heart rate because of direct pressure placed on the extraocular muscles or globe; in the case of orbital floor fractures, entrapment of the inferior rectus can cause pronounced bradycardia, vomiting, syncope, and even asystole, necessitating immediate intervention. Muscle entrapment can also cause persistent postoperative diplopia, ischemic injury and necrosis, or neuropathic injury due to proximity of the infraorbital nerve. In addition, early intervention in cases of significant enophthalmos can prevent long-term posterior displacement of the globe.[9] In the absence of these absolute indications for immediate repair, surgical intervention can be delayed to 2 weeks or later.

Other retrospective studies have identified the average time of repair, associations with postoperative complications, and considerations in the pediatric population. Seifert and colleagues[2] found the average time of intervention to be 6.46 days. In a separate study of oculoplastics versus facial plastics, facial plastics surgeons were more likely to operate after 4 to 7 days, earlier than the oculoplastic surgeons, on average.[12] Seifert and colleagues also found a strong correlation between postoperative complications and an increased time between injury and surgical treatment. However, the investigators noted a caveat to this correlation, as many of their older patients were operated on later due to comorbidities, and these patients had larger defect sizes, which can result in more complications.[2] In the pediatric population, most studies found improved outcomes and faster resolution of diplopia and other symptoms with earlier intervention.[15–17] Jordan and colleagues[18] specifically encouraged immediate surgery after injury in children with the "white-eyed blowout fracture" due to the reduced risk of permanent motility restriction. It is important to identify these specific signs and symptoms for immediate repair and only in the absence of these indications is it prudent to delay reconstruction.

INPATIENT VERSUS OUTPATIENT MANAGEMENT

While determining the need for surgical intervention, the initial evaluation and management of orbital floor fractures should focus on ophthalmic examination and risk of globe injury. Generally, all patients with fractures are instructed to avoid nose-blowing to prevent orbital emphysema and subsequent orbital compartment syndrome. Cold compresses and elevation of the head of the bed are recommended to reduce periorbital edema. In addition, some practitioners encourage the use of steroids for severe periorbital edema and prophylactic antibiotics to prevent orbital cellulitis.[8,9] Further studies are still needed to provide higher quality evidence supporting the efficacy of antibiotics in orbital and upper face fractures.[19,20]

When surgery is indicated, transconjunctival approaches are widely preferred due to better outcomes, such as lack of visible scar, less chance for lid retraction, and no damage to the orbicularis. Even among oculoplastic surgeons and facial plastic surgeons, both groups agreed on the transconjunctival approach.[8,9,12,14] However, this is a less direct approach and has a steeper learning curve to proficiency. In a survey of current management of orbital fractures, Aldekhayel and colleagues[10] found the midlid/infraorbital approaches to be the most common, followed by transconjunctival and subciliary last. The subciliary approach, specifically, has been disfavored in recent years due to increased visibility of the scar and greater risk of cicatricial eyelid malposition and ectropion formation.[9,14] In a 2010 comparative study of different surgical approaches in orbital floor fractures, the subciliary approach resulted in the greatest number of postoperative complications (18.7%), whereas a transconjunctival approach without canthotomy resulted in the least number of complications. However, the investigators recognized the possible need for a subciliary incision when major surgical exposure is needed.[21] A recent meta-analysis compared the complication rate between the transconjunctival and subciliary approaches. The transconjunctival approach resulted in an overall reduced complication rate. However, this approach can often require a secondary surgery, which can increase surgical duration and tissue damage. In comparison, the subciliary approach fully exposes the fracture area, allowing for an easier surgery; yet, this approach carries a higher risk of scarring, muscle damage, ectropion, and other complications.[22] Endoscopic management via transnasal and transantral approaches has also been described. Benefits of these less direct approaches are enhanced visualization, avoidance of adverse effects and scarring to the eyelid, and avoidance of postoperative infraorbital nerve hypesthesia (particularly with the transnasal endoscopic approach). The endoscopic approach also reduces intraoperative blood loss and shortens the hospital stay for patients.[8,23,24] Despite these positive outcomes, endoscopic management of orbital floor fractures has yet to become widely accepted.

Currently, the standard of management is outpatient surgery and postoperative management with the patient able to return home following the surgery. Patients are given pain medications and lubricating ointments, are told to avoid contact sports or nose blowing, and are instructed to call the surgeon with uncontrolled bleeding or vision changes. Follow-up is typically 1 to 2 weeks following surgery.[9] A recent retrospective study compared inpatient versus outpatient management of orbital blowout fractures to evaluate safety outcomes and costs of care. With safer outcomes measured by rate of delayed RBH, the investigators found no data to suggest inpatient orbital blowout repair or overnight monitoring improves outcomes. Inpatient management did not aid in RBH detection in any case nor did overnight admission. In addition, outpatient management was found to be more economical, with reduced total costs of repair.[25] Shew and colleagues had similar findings from their 9-year retrospective study; of the 80 patients, the average length of postsurgical observation was 17 hours. Only one patient presented with RBH 20 hours postoperatively, well past the average length of stay.[26] This aligns with other cases' findings, in which postoperative RBH occurred 29 hours to 10 days later, questioning the benefit of inpatient observation.[27–30] However, studies comparing inpatient versus outpatient surgical management are limited and require further exploration.

INTRAOPERATIVE AND POSTOPERATIVE IMAGING

There has been some debate on the utility of intraoperative and postoperative imaging for orbital floor fractures. Preoperatively, CT is preferred due to its speed and excellent visualization of bony details. CT can be used to determine the size of the fracture, herniation of intraorbital contents, presence of RBH, and injury to the globe. CT can be misleading in cases of pediatric trapdoor fractures; therefore, careful radiologic and clinical evaluation is essential. MRI can be useful for details of the orbital apex; however, metallic foreign body must first be excluded in cases of orbital and facial trauma. x-ray imaging of the orbit has little role in modern trauma evaluation of fractures given the significantly improved anatomic detail on CT.

There is a paucity of literature evaluating the use of intraoperative imaging for orbital fracture reconstruction. Intraoperative CT scans likely have more utility in zygomatico-maxillary complex (ZMC) fractures or in reoperations and may improve surgical outcomes in these specific clinical scenarios. However, intraoperative CT increases operative time as well as exposure to radiation. Jansen and colleagues performed a study of the use of repeat CT scans to assess the position and accuracy of the implant in cadavers. Each reconstruction required a mean of 1.6 scans and significantly improved implant location for orbital floor and medial wall fractures, highlighting the possible utility of intraoperative scans.[31]

Typically, postoperative imaging for orbital floor fractures is obtained secondary to clinical indications, such as limitations in ocular motility, persistent edema, altered mental status, and visual field defects, as supported by the retrospective study conducted by Carpenter and colleagues[32] In the same study, the investigators found postoperative imaging to be more common in orbital floor fractures with ZMC involvement rather than in isolated fractures. Although not useful in asymptomatic patients, postoperative imaging seems to be overused and may be more beneficial and less costly when limited to patients with concerning clinical symptoms. Current guidelines also do not address postoperative imaging, and there would be value in standardizing postoperative imaging guidelines for the management of orbital floor fractures across surgical specialties.[32–34] In situations of post-implant complications such as compartment syndrome, imaging may reveal treatable causes such as hematomas and can identify the source and location of the elevated pressure.[35]

CHOICE OF IMPLANTS

One of the most variable aspects of orbital floor fracture reconstruction is implant type. The ideal implant has several key characteristics: stability and strength to support orbital contents, to retain shape, and ability to be fixated to bony landmarks if necessary. They should be pliable for ease of shaping to the orbit with smooth surfaces to avoid impinging tissues. Biologically, they should be nonallergenic and noncarcinogenic with minimal risks of infection, foreign body reaction, or migration and should resorb at an acceptable pace or be easy to remove. Finally, they should be affordable, readily available, and should not increase complications or risks.[8]

Implants can be classified into autologous, allogenic, and alloplastic sources. Autologous implants (eg, bone from the iliac crest) and allogenic implants (eg, demineralized bone) are rarely used. Alloplastic implants are currently favored for reconstruction of the orbital floor and can be further divided into (1) metallic permanent implants, (2) nonmetallic permanent implants, and (3) bioresorbable implants.

Titanium mesh and vitallium mesh, a titanium alloy, are metallic permanent implants. Titanium implants were originally used for dental and prosthetic implants before becoming incorporated into orbital fracture repair. Titanium is rigid and malleable, providing the ability to reconstruct large defects, and osseointegrates, offering additional strength and stability to the orbital bones.[36] Titanium implants invoke an inflammatory fibrotic response between the implant and orbital tissue, potentially causing diplopia and cicatricial lid changes.[37] Owing to fibrous ingrowth and osseointegration, they are often difficult to remove.[38–45]

Nonmetallic permanent implants consist of materials such as silicone, bioactive glass, porous polyethylene, and nylon. Of the nonmetallic permanent implants, porous polypropylene is a common choice. This is a perforated material that allows for vascular and soft tissue ingrowth, is strong and inert, and is easy to work with. Rates of foreign body reactions, capsule formation, and implant failure also tend to be lower.[46] However, porous polypropylene is radiologically lucent and may be associated with higher rates of infection when exposed to mucosal surfaces.[47–49] Nylon is a nonporous polyamide sheet that has been used for orbital blowout fracture repair since the 1960s. Nylon implants are nonporous materials whose main benefits lie in combination of rigidity and flexibility, range of thickness from 0.05 to 2.0 mm, and ability to be used for combined fractures of the orbital floor and medial orbital wall.[14] Smooth nylon foil implants have also been shown to be safe and effective with low overall complication rates, such as postoperative orbital hemorrhage and infection.[50]

Composite materials, such as titanium mesh embedded in porous polyethylene (Medpor, Synpor), were introduced in the 1980s and are frequently used for orbital floor implants. Titanium provides the strength and ease of contouring in the implants, whereas the porous polyethylene shell prevents orbital adherence and decreased risk of diplopia.[51,52] Composite titanium mesh with porous polyethylene has lower rates of infection and is radiopaque, which is useful for postoperative imaging.

Several resorbable alloplastic implants are also available, with the major benefit of reducing risks of foreign body reactions and long-term consequences. Gelatin film manufactured from denatured collagen has been shown to be effective in reconstruction of defects less than 5 mm with reduced inflammatory responses and implant migration.[52,53] Biodegradable polyglycolic acid is another implant option that has been shown to be easy to work with, malleable once heated, and have minimal migration, with only the postoperative complication of temporary palpebral inflammation.[54] However, for orbital floor defect larger than 1 cm^2, Hollier and colleagues[55] recommended polyglycolic acid not be used due to the complications of enophthalmos and inflammatory reactions requiring the removal of the implants after 6 months. Polydioxanone is a third biodegradable implant material that resorbs after 6 months. There are conflicting reports on the complications and efficacy associated with polydioxanone.[55–59]

Historically, autologous implants such as bone and cartilage were the gold standard due to their strength, rigidity, and revascularization potential with minimal immune reactivity and thus low risk of infection, capsule formation, extrusion, or ocular tethering; however, they have unpredictable resorption rates with differences in resorption between cortical and cancellous bone, leading to an increase in popularity in alloplastic implants in recent years.[9,36,60] Specifically, titanium, porous polyethylene, nylon sheets, or composite implants have become the most popular options. Aldekhayel and colleagues[10] reported that 83% of surgeons preferred using porous polyethylene and titanium implants compared with only 4% still using autologous bone implants. In their comparison of trends between oculofacial surgeons and facial plastic surgeons, Cohen and colleagues[12] found that both groups preferred to use porous polyethylene and titanium combination implants or nylon implants. Bioresorbable implants are an alternative option in select cases. Overall, trends indicate a move away from autologous toward alloplastic materials, yet the identification of the most ideal alloplastic implant remains controversial.

SUMMARY

Orbital floor fractures remain a common complication of facial trauma. Ophthalmic examination and evaluation of the globe are an essential first step in the management of orbital fractures. Indications for repair include entrapment of orbital tissue, large fracture defects with herniation of orbital contents, persistent diplopia, and clinically significant enophthalmos. The transconjunctival approach for surgical repair is preferred to reduce the risk of cicatricial lid malposition. There is currently no compelling evidence supporting inpatient management following fracture repair or the use of intraoperative CT in isolated primary orbital floor fractures. Postoperative CT should be reserved for cases with specific postoperative clinical indications. Alloplastic implant materials are widely preferred, and implant choice remains controversial and variable between surgeons based on training and expertise.

CLINICS CARE POINTS

- Examination is essential for the evaluation of orbital floor fractures to ensure surgical intervention is indicated.
- In the absence of the oculocardiac reflex and tissue entrapment, surgical intervention should be delayed for 1 to 2 weeks to allow for reduction in edema and accurate assessment of need for repair.
- Current evidence suggests outpatient surgical management is adequate for orbital floor fractures with minimal additional benefit of inpatient management.
- Among the many surgical approaches for correction, the transconjunctival approach offers better outcomes, less scarring, and fewer risks.
- Postoperative imaging tends to be overused and should be limited to patients with post-implant complications or concerning symptoms.

FUNDING

No funding or sponsorship was received for this study or publication of this article.

DISCLOSURES

The authors have no commercial or financial conflicts of interest.

REFERENCES

1. Chiang E, Saadat LV, Spitz JA, et al. Etiology of orbital fractures at a level i trauma center in a large metropolitan City. Taiwan J Ophthalmol 2016;6(1):26–31.
2. Seifert LB, Mainka T, Herrera-Vizcaino C, et al. Orbital floor fractures: epidemiology and outcomes of 1594 reconstructions. Eur J Trauma Emerg Surg 2022; 48(2):1427–36.
3. Luibil N, Lopez MJ and Patel BC. Anatomy, Head and neck, orbit. In: StatPearls [Internet]. Treasure Island (FL), 2023, StatPearls Publishing.
4. Hammer B. Orbital fractures: diagnosis, operative treatment, secondary corrections. Boston, MA: Hogrefe & Huber Publishers; 1995.
5. Parameswaran A, Marimuthu M, Panwar S, et al. Orbital fractures. Oral and maxillofacial Surgery for the clinician. Singapore: Springer Nature Singapore; 2021. p. 1201–50.
6. King EF, Samuel E. Fractures of the orbit. Trans Ophthalmol Soc U K 1944;64: 134–53.
7. Le Fort R. Etude Experimentale sur les Fractures de la Machoire Superieure. Revue de Chirurgie de Paris 1901;23:208–479.

8. Joseph J, Glavas IP. Orbital fractures: a review. Clin Ophthalmol 2011;5:95.

9. Boyette J, Pemberton J, Bonilla-Velez J. Management of orbital rractures: challenges and solutions. Clin Ophthalmol 2015;9:2127.

10. Aldekhayel S, Aljaaly H, Fouda-Neel O, et al. Evolving trends in the management of orbital floor fractures. J Craniofac Surg 2014;25(1):258–61.

11. Basta MN, Rao V, Roussel LO, et al. Refining indications for orbital floor fracture reconstruction: a risk-stratification tool predicting symptom development and need for surgery. Plast Reconstr Surg 2021;148(3):606–15.

12. Cohen LM, Shaye DA, Yoon MK. Isolated orbital floor fracture management: a survey and comparison of American oculofacial and facial plastic surgeon preferences. Craniomaxillofacial Trauma Reconstr 2019;12(2):112–21.

13. Christensen BJ, Zaid W. Inaugural survey on practice patterns of orbital floor fractures for american oral and maxillofacial surgeons. J Oral Maxillofac Surg 2016; 74(1):105–22.

14. Grob S, Yonkers M, Tao J. Orbital fracture repair. Semin Plast Surg 2017;31(01): 031–9.

15. Egbert JE, May K, Kersten RC, et al. Pediatric orbital floor fracture. Ophthalmol Times 2000;107(10):1875–9.

16. Grant JH, Patrinely JR, Weiss AH, et al. Trapdoor fracture of the orbit in a pediatric population. Plast Reconstr Surg 2002;109(2):482–9.

17. Wei LA, Durairaj VD. Pediatric orbital floor fractures. J Am Assoc Pediatr Ophthalmol Strabismus 2011;15(2):173–80.

18. Jordan DR, Allen LH, White J, et al. Intervention within days for some orbital floor fractures. Ophthal Plast Reconstr Surg 1998;14(6):379–90.

19. Mundinger GS, Borsuk DE, Okhah Z, et al. Antibiotics and facial fractures: evidence-based recommendations compared with experience-based practice. Craniomaxillofacial Trauma Reconstr 2015;8(1):64–78.

20. Reiss B, Rajjoub L, Mansour T, et al. Antibiotic prophylaxis in orbital fractures. Open Ophthalmol J 2017;11(1):11–6.

21. Salgarelli AC, Bellini P, Landini B, et al. A Comparative study of different approaches in the treatment of orbital trauma: an experience based on 274 cases. Oral Maxillofac Surg 2010;14(1):23–7.

22. Zhang J, He X, Qi Y, et al. The better surgical timing and approach for orbital fracture: a systematic review and meta-analysis. Ann Transl Med 2022;10(10):564.

23. Cheong EC, Chen CT, Chen YR. Endoscopic management of orbital floor fractures. Facial Plast Surg 2009;25(01):008–16.

24. Ikeda K, Suzuki H, Oshima T, et al. Endoscopic endonasal repair of orbital floor fracture. Arch Otolaryngol Head Neck Surg 1999;125(1):59.

25. Bregman JA, Vakharia KT, Idowu OO, et al. Outpatient surgical management of orbital blowout fractures. Craniomaxillofacial Trauma Reconstr 2019;12(3): 205–10.

26. Shew M, Carlisle MP, Lu G, et al. Surgical treatment of orbital blowout fractures: complications and postoperative care patterns. Craniomaxillofacial Trauma Reconstr 2016;9(4):299–304.

27. Nicholson DH, Guzak SV. Visual loss complicating repair of orbital floor fractures. Arch Ophthalmol 1971;86(4):369–75.

28. Ord RA. Post-operative retrobulbar haemorrhage and blindness complicating trauma surgery. Br J Oral Maxillofac Surg 1981;19(3):202–7.

29. Cheon JS, Seo BN, Yang JY, et al. Retrobulbar hematoma in blow-out fracture after open reduction. Arch Plast Surg 2013;40(04):445–9.

30. Girotto JA, Gamble WB, Robertson B, et al. Blindness after reduction of facial fractures. Plast Reconstr Surg 1998;102(6):1821–34.
31. Jansen J, Schreurs R, Dubois L, et al. Intraoperative imaging in orbital reconstruction: how does it affect the position of the implant? Br J Oral Maxillofac Surg 2020;58(7):801–6.
32. Carpenter D, Shammas R, Honeybrook A, et al. The role of postoperative imaging after orbital floor fracture repair. Craniomaxillofacial Trauma Reconstr 2018;11(2):96–101.
33. Gart MS, Gosain AK. Evidence-based medicine. Plast Reconstr Surg 2014;134(6):1345–55.
34. Burnstine MA. Clinical recommendations for repair of isolated orbital floor fractures. Ophthalmol Times 2002;109(7):1207–10.
35. Lin KY, Ngai P, Echegoyen JC, et al. Imaging in orbital trauma. Saudi J Ophthalmol 2012;26(4):427–32.
36. Mok D, Lessard L, Cordoba C, et al. A review of materials currently used in orbital floor reconstruction. Can J Plast Surg 2004;12(3):134–40.
37. Lee HB, Nunery WR. Orbital adherence syndrome secondary to titanium implant. Material. Ophthal Plast Reconstr Surg 2009;25:33–6.
38. Schubert W, Gear AJL, Lee C, et al. Incorporation of titanium mesh in orbital and midface reconstruction. Plast Reconstr Surg 2002;110(4):1022–30.
39. Rubin PJ, Yaremchuk MJ. Complications and toxicities of implantable biomaterials used in facial reconstructive and aesthetic surgery: a comprehensive review of the literature. Plast Reconstr Surg 1997;100(5):1336–53.
40. Avashia YJ, Sastry A, Fan KL, et al. Materials used for reconstruction after orbital floor fracture. J Craniofac Surg 2012;23(7):S49–55.
41. Schlittler F, Vig N, Burkhard JP, et al. What are the limitations of the non-patient-specific implant in titanium reconstruction of the orbit? Br J Oral Maxillofac Surg 2020;58(9):e80–5.
42. Haug RH, Nuveen E, Bredbenner T. An evaluation of the support provided by common internal orbital reconstruction materials. J Oral Maxillofac Surg 1999;57(5):564–70.
43. Laxenaire A, Lévy J, Blanchard P, et al. Complications of silastic implants used in orbital repair. Rev Stomatol Chir Maxillofac 1997;98(Suppl 1):96–9.
44. Aitasalo K, Kinnunen I, Palmgren J, et al. Repair of orbital floor fractures with bioactive glass implants. J Oral Maxillofac Surg 2001;59(12):1390–5.
45. Zide MF. Late posttraumatic enophthalmos corrected by dense hydroxylapatite blocks. J Oral Maxillofac Surg 1986;44(10):804–6.
46. Gunarajah DR, Samman N. Biomaterials for repair of orbital floor blowout fractures: a systematic review. J Oral Maxillofac Surg 2013;71(3):550–70.
47. Villarreal PM, Monje F, Morillo AJ, et al. Porous polyethylene implants in orbital floor reconstruction. Plast Reconstr Surg 2002;109(3):877–85.
48. Karesh JW, Dresner SC. High-density porous polyethylene (medpor) as a successful anophthalmic socket implant. Ophthalmol Times 1994;101(10):1688–95 [discussion: 1695-6].
49. Timoney PJ, Clark JD, Frederick PA, et al. Foreign body granuloma following orbital reconstruction with porous polyethylene. Ophthal Plast Reconstr Surg 2016;32(6):e137–8.
50. Park DJJ, Garibaldi DC, Lliff NT, et al. Smooth nylon foil (SupraFOIL) orbital implants in orbital fractures: a case series of 181 patients. Ophthal Plast Reconstr Surg 2008;24(4):266–70.

51. Garibaldi DC, Iliff NT, Grant MP, et al. Use of porous polyethylene with embedded titanium in orbital reconstruction: a review of 106 patients. Ophthal Plast Reconstr Surg 2007;23:439–44.
52. Zhang L, Fay A. Composite implants in oculoplastic surgery. Semin Ophthalmol 2010;25:303–8.
53. Parkin JL, Stevens MH, Stringham JC. Absorbable gelatin film versus silicone rubber sheeting in orbital fracture treatment. Laryngoscope 1987;97(1):1–3.
54. Mermer RW, Orban RE. Repair of orbital floor fractures with absorbable gelatin film. J Craniomaxillofac Trauma 1995;1(4):30–4.
55. Hollier LH, Rogers N, Berzin E, et al. Resorbable mesh in the treatment of orbital floor fractures. J Craniofac Surg 2001;12(3):242–6.
56. Piotrowski WP, Mayer-Zuchi U. The use of polyglactin 910-polydioxanon in the treatment of defects of the orbital roof. J Oral Maxillofac Surg 1999;57(11): 1301–5.
57. Baumann A, Burggasser G, Gauss N, et al. Orbital floor reconstruction with an alloplastic resorbable polydioxanone sheet. Int J Oral Maxillofac Surg 2002; 31(4):367–73.
58. Kontio R, Suuronen R, Salonen O, et al. Effectiveness of operative treatment of internal orbital wall fracture with polydioxanone implant. Int J Oral Maxillofac Surg 2001;30(4):278–85.
59. Jank S, Emshoff R, Schuchter B, et al. Orbital floor reconstruction with flexible ethisorb patches: a retrospective long-term follow-up study. Oral Surg Oral Med Oral Pathol Oral Radiol Endod 2003;95(1):16–22.
60. Dubois L, Steenen SA, Gooris PJJ, et al. Controversies in orbital reconstruction— III. Biomaterials for orbital reconstruction: a review with clinical recommendations. Int J Oral Maxillofac Surg 2016;45(1):41–50.

Applications of Maxillomandibular Fixation, Occlusal Guidance, and Jaw Physiotherapy in the Management of Fractures of the Mandible

Daniel J. Meara, MS, MD, DMD, MHCDS[a,b],*

KEYWORDS

- Mandible • Fractures • Occlusion • Maxillomandibular fixation • Elastic guidance
- Jaw physiotherapy

KEY POINTS

- The goal of mandibular fracture management is to restore form and function.
- Maxillomandibular fixation, elastic occlusal guidance, and postoperative physiotherapy are essential elements to optimizing outcomes.
- Bone healing, an idealized occlusion, and normal JROM signal success via the restoration of form and function.

DEFINITIONS

Occlusion is the contact between the maxillary and mandibular teeth.

Occlusal guidance is comprised of movements of the mandible as a result of tooth contact with the maxillary dentition.

Maxillomandibular fixation involves immobilizing the mobile mandible and aligning mandibular and maxillary teeth with tight fixation.

With crossbite, maxillary teeth are medial/lingual to the mandibular teeth in the anterior or posterior areas, or both.

An overjet is horizontal projection of the anterior maxillary teeth in-relation to the mandibular anterior teeth.

[a] Oral and Maxillofacial Surgery, Department of Oral and Maxillofacial Surgery & Hospital Dentistry, Christiana Care Health System, Wilmington, DE, USA; [b] Affiliate Faculty, Department of Physical Therapy, University of Delaware, Newark, DE, USA
* Oral and Maxillofacial Surgery, Department of Oral and Maxillofacial Surgery & Hospital Dentistry, Christiana Care Health System, Wilmington, DE.
E-mail address: dmeara@christianacare.org

Otolaryngol Clin N Am 56 (2023) 1113–1123
https://doi.org/10.1016/j.otc.2023.07.001
0030-6665/23/© 2023 Elsevier Inc. All rights reserved.

oto.theclinics.com

An overbite is vertical projection of the anterior maxillary teeth in-relation to the mandibular anterior teeth.

An open bite is the relationship of teeth in, which the maxillary teeth and mandibular teeth do not make contact.

CLASSIFICATION OF OCCLUSION

The Edward angle of classification is the gold standard for the classification of dental occlusion, as it relates to the permanent dentition.[1]

Normal Occlusion

For normal occlusion, the mesiobuccal cusp of the upper maxillary first molar occludes in the buccal groove of the mandibular first molar (**Fig. 1**). The maxillary canine occludes with the distal half of the mandibular canine and the mesial half of the mandibular first premolar.

Malocclusions are determined by the occlusal relationship of the first molars, and 3 types exist. Canine relationships can also be a point of reference for the occlusal relationship.

Class I

Class I occlusions are similar to normal occlusions except that there is an incorrect occlusion because of misaligned teeth, crowding, and rotations of the teeth despite a normal first molar relationship.

Class II

In Class II occlusions, the molar occlusal relationship is one in which the mesiobuccal cusp of the maxillary first molar is anterior to the buccal groove of the mandibular first molar (**Fig. 2**).

The maxillary canine occlusal relationship is anterior to the mandibular canine.

Retrognathia is a convex face profile resulting from a mandible that is too small or maxilla that is too large, or a combination of both.

Class II malocclusion has two subtypes, relating to the anterior teeth (**Fig. 3**).

Class II division 1
The molar relationships are like that of class II, and the maxillary anterior teeth are protruded, creating a large overjet.

Class II division 2
The molar relationships are class II, where the maxillary central incisors are retroclined, creating a deep overbite.

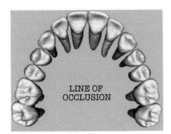
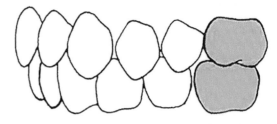

Fig. 1. Normal occlusion.

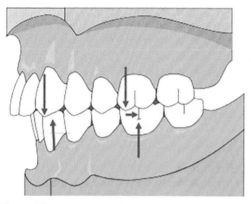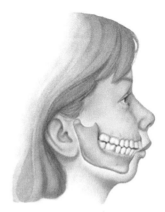

Fig. 2. Class II malocclusion.

Class II Division 1	Class II Division 2
Upper incisors are **PROCLINED**	Upper central incisors show **LINGUAL INCLINATION** and may be **OVERLAPPED** by upper lateral incisors
Excessive **OVERJET** and **DEEP OVERBITE**	**DEEP OVERBITE**
V-shped upper arch, **NARROW** in canine region **BROAD** between molars	**BROAD** upper arch (usually)
SHORTER UPPER LIP - failure in anterior lip closure	**NORMAL UPPER LIP** and lip seal **DEEP MENTAL GROOVE**
Mandible may be deficient and chin **UNDERDEVELOPED**	Mandible is of a **GOOD SIZE**

Fig. 3. Class II malocclusion, divisions 1 and 2.

Class III

In class III occlusion, the molar occlusal relationship is one in which the mesiobuccal cusp of the maxillary first molar is posterior to the buccal groove of the mandibular first molar (**Fig. 4**).

The mesial surface of the maxillary canine is posterior to the distal surface of the mandibular canine and the mandibular incisors are in crossbite.

There may be concave face profile resulting from a mandible that is too large or a maxilla that is too small, or a combination of both.

GOALS–WHY IS THIS IMPORTANT?

Mandible fractures require bony reduction and immobilization for proper bone healing, but the mandible is unique as related to the other facial bones, as it is a mobile bone that rotates and translates, and it must align with the opposing maxilla. Thus, maxillo-mandibular fixation (MMF), even if transient, is required for almost all cases to align the dental arches before any application of fixation.[2] The key concept is that the mandible and maxilla must be ideally aligned via the dentition before fixation of any type, because, if fixation occurs without alignment, then the risk of an iatrogenic malocclusion is significant, and the resultant patient outcomes will be compromised, despite successful bony healing. Exceptions occur in cases in which postinjury occlusion is maintained, and the patient does not require any surgical intervention or occlusal guidance, such as in condylar head fractures or greenstick fractures.

CHALLENGES

Challenges with properly employing maxillomandibular fixation in mandible fractures include poor dentition, missing dentition, mixed dentition in pediatric patients, and dentofacial deformities. Issues such as these create the inability to assure stable and secure alignment between the arches is achieved before application of fixation. Specifically, poor dentition and missing dentition cases often result in sliding arches and unstable MMF. Cases with missing dentition, especially missing posterior dentition, are prone to unstable MMF, and with no posterior dental points of contact, the mandible can be over-rotated in a clockwise direction. Patients with dentofacial deformities often create a challenge, as it can be unclear as to what type of occlusion is the

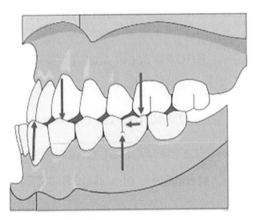
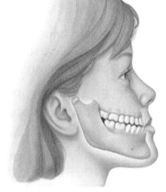

Fig. 4. Class III malocclusion.

patient's baseline occlusal scheme. For instance, in a class III malocclusion patient, the surgeon must avoid the desire to create a normal class I occlusion for the patient, as this will not be possible, especially if proper bony reduction is achieved. Another special group is comprised of fully edentulous patients, those with no remaining teeth. In this group, establishing an occlusion is often immaterial, but in patients with denture teeth, aligning the maxillary and mandibular dentures before fixation assures that pre-morbid fit is maintained. Further, denture teeth can facilitate the surgery, by preventing mandibular movement and helping maintain bony reduction before the application of fixation. Also, in the completely edentulous patient without denture teeth, Gunning splints, designed by Gunning in the 1960s, are an option.

PITFALLS

As mandibular fracture repair is not solely about achieving healing of the fractures bone, failure to understand and employ MMF can result in suboptimal outcomes by creating a new occlusion, likely to be a malocclusion that the patient will likely find problematic. Also, if the mandibular condyle is overseated, in class III cases, the patient may develop temporomandibular joint symptoms and in class II cases, the patient is likely to develop an anterior open bite once MMF is released and the mandibular condyles freely rotate back into the glenoid fossa.

TIPS AND TRICKS

Achieving MMF is foundational in the proper repair of almost all mandible fractures. Success is likely when the surgical team understands the concept of dental occlusion, applies it correctly to each case, and uses tricks of the trade as warranted to facilitate optimal occlusal outcomes in patients who present challenges in achieving premorbid occlusion. Wear facets, patient and family input, existing pictures of the patient smiling tooth, and orthodontic records are tools to optimized MMF.

Wear facets are surface changes to the tooth enamel caused by tooth-to-tooth contact and habits such as grinding over many years (**Fig. 5**). The tooth enamel changes create facets, in which the opposing teeth easily align, and these relationships facilitate proper MMF.

Patient and family input is another means to understand the patient's premorbid occlusion. Input before surgery can allay concerns around the patient's occlusal scheme, especially in complex fractures. As there is typically a malocclusion as a result of the mandible fracture, clinical examination determination of the patient's

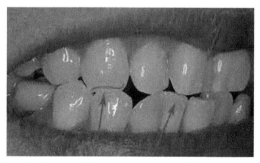

Fig. 5. Dental attrition. (*Red arrows*) demonstrate areas of dental attrition that suggest how the dental arches should align, based on a predictable pattern of tooth wear from contact.

baseline occlusion is often impossible, and thus, input from the patient or the family, when the patient is incapacitated, can facilitate MMF.

Pictures of the patient smiling also help determine a patient's premorbid occlusion. For example, a family photo may demonstrate that the patient is prognathic and has a class III malocclusion.

Lastly, orthodontic records can occasionally be obtained preoperatively; if the patient has a relatively recent history of orthodontic treatment, the clinical records and radiographs should define the patient's occlusion.

TOOLS FOR MAXILLOMANDIBULAR FIXATION APPLICATION
Erich Arch Bars

Erich arch bars are the historic norm for employing MMF (**Fig. 6**A). The arch bars are stainless steel, easily adapted, and low profile. Each bar is typically attached from at least first molar to first molar, with stainless steel interdental wires around each tooth to secure the bar. Additional advantages include low cost and avoidance of tooth roots and other vital structures such as the mental nerve. Disadvantages include more potential for surgical team iatrogenic finger skin punctures, potential for luxation of teeth, and increased time of application compared with hybrid or bone-anchored arch bars.

Hybrid Arch Bars

Hybrid arch bars are a mix conceptually of Erich arch bars and intermaxillary fixation (IMF) screws (**Fig. 6**B). Specifically, the hybrid arch bars are bone anchored with screws that secure the titanium bar to the dental arch. Advantages include great stability of the bar and ability to tightly cinch the opposing arches into a tight MMF. Further advantages include ease and reduced time of application. Disadvantages include increased cost and mucosal and gingival irritation by the rigid lugs projecting from the bar. Also, risk of tooth root injury requires proper screw length and evaluation of the patient's imaging to assess for bony windows between roots to place bar fixation screws.

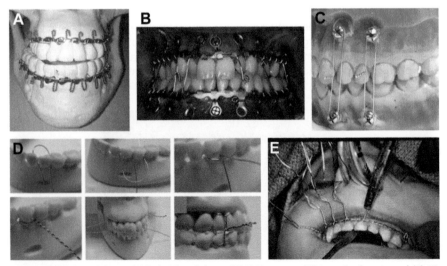

Fig. 6. (A) Erich arch bars, (B) hybrid arch bars, (C) IMF screws, (D) Ivy wire loops, and (E) Risdon wire.

Intermaxillary Fixation Screws

IMF screws are individual screws placed into bone, bilaterally in the oral cavity, to allow for wire loops from mandibular to maxillary opposing screws to achieved MMF (**Fig. 6**C). Typically, these screws are best for cases with a full dentition. Advantages include ease of application, reduced time of placement, and reduced impact on gingival tissues that can be seen with arch bars. Disadvantages include risk for injury to the roots of teeth and vital structures such as the mental nerve foramen and irritation of the lips and cheeks due to frictional irritation. Further, IMF screws provide limited occlusal elastic guidance postoperatively.

Ivy Loops

Ivy loops are stainless steel wires typically applied bilaterally to the maxillary and mandibular arches to create buccal loops that allow for MMF with wires or elastics, although this method is often not as secure and reliable in cases of compromised dentition or for longer periods of MMF (**Fig. 6**D). Advantages include ease of application, low cost, patient tolerance, and use in pediatric patients with mixed dentition. Disadvantages include less rigid MMF.

Risdon Wire for Pediatrics

The Risdon wire is an arch bar created by twisting bilateral wires into an arch bar that is then secured around the primary dentition or mixed dentition (**Fig. 6**E). This technique allows adaptation to the pediatric dental arch and primary teeth or mixed dentition, which can be difficult with a traditional arch bar. Further, in the pediatric patient with primary or mixed dentition, IMF screws or hybrid arch bars are contraindicated because of the likelihood of damaging the developing permanent dentition.

TECHNIQUE HIGHLIGHTS
Cost

Contemporary studies have compared the total costs of Erich arch bars versus bone-borne arch bars, and as a result of operating room time saved with bone-borne arch bars, the total cost of care is similar, despite the significantly increased cost of titanium bone-borne hybrid arch bars.[3]

Time

Erich arch bars take about 15 minutes per arch to apply, whereas hybrid arch bars take about 5 minutes per arch.

Dentition

At a minimum, a tripod occlusion is necessary to achieve a stable and accurate MMF. As a general rule, the fewer teeth that a patient has means, the more extensive the MMF device, meaning that in a full dentition, all options are available to the surgeon for MMF. In partial edentulism or poor dentition cases, an Erich arch bar or bone-borne arch bar is best to achieve the best possible alignment of the dental arches before application of fixation.

Fracture Type

The fracture type plays a role in determining the type of MMF device to be employed. For instance, a minimal or nondisplaced mandibular fracture is amendable to most MMF techniques. In contrast, an unfavorable fracture with displacement or with multiple mandibular fractures or associated maxillary fractures will require an arch bar to achieve stable MMF.

Pearls

In displaced or mobile mandibular fractures, it is important to understand that application of an arch bar will create mandibular arch stability but can make ideal fracture segment reduction more challenging. Thus, avoidance of overtightening of the arch bar will allow for fracture segment reduction and idealization of occlusion.

Avoid Injuries

Protection of the surgical team during the application of MMF devices is most challenging with Erich arch bars, as many individual wires need to be applied, and finger stick injuries can easily occur. To minimize the risk, the surgical team should consider only placing 1 circumdental wire at a time, in lieu of having multiple wires placed before cutting the wire ends. Hybrid arch bars or IMF screws minimize this issue.

Avoid Vital Structures

When employing IMF screws or hybrid bone-borne arch bars, it is important to review the patient's radiographs to assess root position and other key anatomical structures such as the maxillary sinus, nasal floor, and the inferior alveolar nerve/mental nerve foramen. Studies have repeatedly demonstrated the ability of IMF and hybrid arch bar screws to damage tooth roots. As a general rule, initial placement should be between roots and at or slightly below the mucogingival junction. However, anterior screw placement often needs to be placed more inferior, as the central incisor teeth are easily displaced by the screw penetration into the thin adjacent bone.

The Combination Technique

Placement of an IMF screw or hybrid arch bar screw into the tissues adjacent to the fracture site can be problematic, obscuring visualization or application of fixation plates. In such situations, a combination technique can be employed at the fracture site, by applying wires around the hybrid arch bar only at the fracture site, ensuring that the arch bar area is low profile, especially in cases in which the hybrid arch bar has loops projecting down from the bar.

EXCEPTIONS
Panfacial Fractures

Panfacial fractures can present a unique situation that may preclude the concept of MMF, as there is generally no stable frame of reference in either the mandible or maxilla. With the bottom-up approach to facial reconstruction in panfacial fractures, the mandible is then idealized via a bony reduction, and the mandible is then the stable frame of reference for the remaining reconstruction.

Edentulism, Complete

In patients who are completely edentulous, MMF may not be part of the mandibular fracture repair, unless the patient has denture teeth or a Gunning splint. For example, Gunning splints can be designed with embedded hooks to facilitate MMF (**Fig. 7**).

IMPLICATIONS

If mandibular bony fixation occurs without assuring proper occlusion with MMF, a malocclusion may be created that is permanent. The result of a persistent malocclusion can be patient dissatisfaction and the development of a temporomandibular joint (TMJ) disorder.

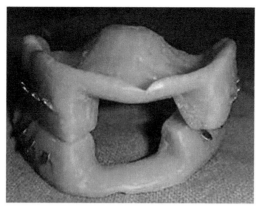

Fig. 7. Gunning splints.

SURGICAL CORRECTION
Orthognathic Surgery and Temporomandibular Joint

Procedures to address a postrepair malocclusion include orthognathic surgery and in cases of mandibular fractures that include the condyle, TMJ total joint replacement.

PHYSIOTHERAPY AND POSTOPERATIVE MANAGEMENT

Mandibular fracture repair and management does not end with surgery. Postoperative care is often critical to successful healing and the complete return to form and function. Management considerations in the postoperative period include: need for MMF or elastic occlusal guidance, diet restrictions, jaw range of motion exercises, and oral wound care/hygiene.

Maxillomandibular Fixation, Postoperative

Postoperative MMF is employed for various reasons, including tenuous fixation due to poor bone stock or concerns over patient compliance with postoperative diet and function.

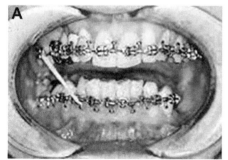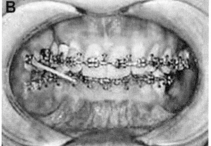

Fig. 8. Elastic guidance to guide occlusion and jaw motion. (*A*) class iii type of elastic on right side to create desired forces to facilitate occlusal goals. technique differs based on desired occlusal outcome and postoperative forces of muscles of mastication. (*B*) idealized postoperative occlusion facilitated by elastic guidance and muscle training.

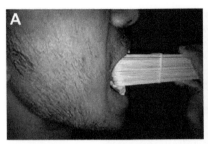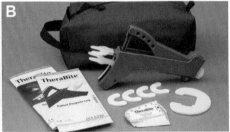

Fig. 9. (A) Tongue depressor sticks and (B) Therabyte device for JROM exercises.

Elastic Guidance

More commonly, postoperative occlusal guidance is employed in the postoperative period to retrain the muscles of mastication and to avoid dysfunctional movements, so as to reinforce the desired occlusion (**Fig. 8**). Further, utilization of elastics can control range of motion and thereby minimize diet indiscretions such as an immediate return to a regular diet by the patient, when a soft diet is prescribed.

Jaw Range of Motion

Home physiotherapy and jaw range of motion (JROM) exercises are indicated at about 6 weeks postoperatively as bony union is occurring and any early postoperative issues have been addressed.[4] Tongue blades are a simple approach to increasing JROM (**Fig. 9**A, B). Specifically, with this technique, the patient's maximal incisal opening is measured, and the exact number of tongue blades to achieve that maximal incisional opening (MIO) is determined. The tongues blades are grouped together and placed between the upper and lower incisors. The patient is instructed to add a new tongue blade the group every 2 to 3 days as long as there is no significant increase in pain with the addition. This process continues until the patient has achieved a normal MIO, approximately 40 mm, which is approximately 3 finger breadths.

Closed reduction/treatment, in which MMF is employed postoperatively for 6 weeks may require a more intensive rehabilitation physiotherapy to restore JROM. In this case, a Therabyte device can be instituted for daily jaw stretching, as is often employed for TMJ patients (see **Fig. 8**). In more recalcitrant cases of reduced postoperative JROM, a referral to physical therapy may be warranted to accelerate the progress towards a return to normal JROM.

SUMMARY

The goal of mandibular fracture management is to restore form and function. MMF, elastic occlusal guidance, and postoperative physiotherapy are essential elements to optimizing outcomes. Specifically, success is not defined by bone healing alone, as in mandible fractures, restoration of premorbid occlusion is paramount. Thus, an expert understanding of occlusion, coupled with the application of maxillomandibular techniques to achieve bony reduction with idealized dental occlusion, is required for the proper management of mandible fractures. Postoperatively, complete recovery often initially requires elastic occlusal guidance followed by JROM physiotherapy. Bone healing, an idealized occlusion, and normal JROM signal success via the restoration of form and function.

CLINICS CARE POINTS

- The mandible and maxilla must be ideally aligned via the dentition before fixation of any type, because, if fixation occurs without alignment, then the risk of an iatrogenic malocclusion is significant.
- Challenges with properly employing maxillomandibular fixation in mandible fractures include poor dentition, missing dentition, mixed dentition in pediatric patients, and dentofacial deformities.
- Patients with dentofacial deformities often create a challenge, as it can be unclear as to what type of occlusion is the patient's baseline occlusal scheme.
- Mandibular fracture repair is not solely about achieving healing of the fractures bone, failure to understand and employ MMF can result in suboptimal outcomes by creating a new occlusion, likely to be a malocclusion.
- Wear facets, patient and family input, existing pictures of the patient smiling tooth, and orthodontic records are tools to optimized MMF.
- Displaced or mobile mandibular fractures, it is important to understand that application of an arch bar will create mandibular arch stability but can make ideal fracture segment reduction more challenging.
- Management considerations in the postoperative period include: need for MMF or elastic occlusal guidance, diet restrictions, jaw range of motion exercises, and oral wound care/hygiene.
- Postoperative occlusal guidance is employed in the postoperative period to retrain the muscles of mastication and to avoid dysfunctional movements, so as to reinforce the desired occlusion.
- Closed reduction/treatment, in which MMF is employed postoperatively for 6 weeks may require a more intensive rehabilitation physiotherapy to restore JROM.

REFERENCES

1. *Angle classification of malocclusion*, 2015, Dentodontics.com. Available at: https://dentodontics.com/2015/09/09/angles-classification-of-malocclusion/.
2. Maxillomandibular Fixation. Available at: https://surgeryreference.aofoundation.org/cmf/basic-technique/maxillomandibular-fixation-mmf-bone-supported-devices.
3. King BJ, Christensen BJ. Hybrid arch bars reduce placement time and glove perforations compared with erich arch bars during the application of intermaxillary fixation: a randomized controlled trial. J Oral Maxillofac Surg 2019;77:1228.e1–8.
4. Hatwar VA, Kulkarni CA, Patil S. Rehabilitation and management of complex multiple para-symphysis mandible fracture: a case report. Cureus 2022;14(11): e31180.

Applications of Preoperative and Intraoperative Technologies for Complex Primary and Secondary Facial Trauma Reconstruction

Alexandrea Kim, MD, Anthony Botros, MD,
Oswaldo A. Henriquez, MD*

KEYWORDS

- Computed tomography • Intraoperative imaging • Craniofacial trauma
- Computer-assisted surgery • Virtual planning • Patient-specific implants

KEY POINTS

- The use of technology in the preoperative and intraoperative phases in the management of complex and secondary maxillofacial reconstruction can improve surgical outcomes.
- Most of the literature that supports the use of these technologies is of a low level of evidence.
- Although these technologies may facilitate and improve outcomes in complex and secondary maxillofacial reconstruction, they do not replace the need for adequate surgical training and surgical planning.

INTRODUCTION

Advancements in the management of maxillofacial trauma have always been linked to the evolution of medical technology. The development of titanium plates for fixation, the advent of computed tomography (CT), and the creation of polymers such as polyetheretherketone (PEEK) for the design of patient-specific implants, are a few examples of how technology has shaped how one approaches the care of patients with maxillofacial trauma.

Department of Otolaryngology-Head & Neck Surgery, Emory University School of Medicine, Atlanta, GA, USA
* Corresponding author. Department of Otolaryngology-Head & Neck Surgery, Emory University School of Medicine, 9th Floor, Medical Office Tower 550 Peachtree Street NE, Atlanta, GA 30308.
E-mail address: oswaldohenriquezaa@gmail.com

Otolaryngol Clin N Am 56 (2023) 1125–1136
https://doi.org/10.1016/j.otc.2023.07.002
0030-6665/23/© 2023 Elsevier Inc. All rights reserved.

For many years it has been recognized that proper imaging is imperative for the diagnosis and treatment plan of injuries of maxillofacial injuries. As the resolution of CT has become greater, so has sensitivity and specificity to diagnosed maxillofacial fractures.[1,2] These improvements in CT have led to some amazing applications in the preoperative and intraoperative phases in the management of maxillofacial trauma such as 3-dimensional imaging and printing/modeling, patient-specific implants, virtual planning, and computer-assisted surgery.

HIGH-DEFINITION COMPUTED TOMOGRAPHY (THREE-DIMENSIONAL MODELING)

The establishment of 3-dimensional rendered models in facial trauma over the years has allowed for the surgeon to shift the preparation and treatment of facial trauma. Before 3-dimensional CT, and currently in areas lacking ready access to CT technology, conventional radiology and ultrasonography were and are widely used along the midface and mandible to diagnose fractures. In a study comparing the utility of the 2 modalities, the specificity and sensitivity of detecting fractures via ultrasound were 100% and 91%, respectively, with the worst specificity and the symphysis of the mandible.[3] The sensitivity dropped to 84.6% in the presence of a hematoma. This is compared with 100% sensitivity and specificity when using CT as a diagnostic modality. In the case of comparing the use of conventional radiographs with CT, studies have shown a significant superiority of diagnoses on CT.[4] Although imaging modalities such as ultrasound and conventional radiographs remain an affordable option for diagnosing fractures in the low-income setting, as well as in the pediatric population where limiting radiation exposure is desired, access to CT imaging is the gold standard for definitively detecting facial fractures.

3-dimensional CT modeling goes beyond just detecting facial fractures, however. This innovative technology has allowed the surgeon to simulate the planned surgery ahead of time with excellent precision, thus reducing surgical operative time and optimizing aesthetic and functional outcomes.[5] The availability of excellent 3-dimensional imaging rendering is obtained with 0.625 mm (about 0.02 in) CT image slices (typically requiring 250–350 image slices to capture the entirety of the face). The result of this is

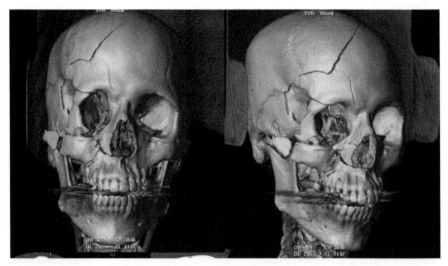

Fig. 1. An example of a 3-dimensional rendering of a patient with midface fractures.

an excellent visualization of the mandibular and midface structures (**Fig. 1**). The 3-dimensional CT can also be used to visualize vascularity in head and neck reconstruction cases.

VIRTUAL SURGICAL PLANNING

Virtual surgical planning (VSP) is the process of planning and rehearsing a surgical procedure on computer models. VSP has been combined with 3-dimensional printing technology to improve surgical efficiency and precision through the production of 3-dimensional surgical models, guides, and implants.[6,7] Both VSP and 3-dimensional models can be used to place the ideal amount, shape, and dimensions of material needed for maxillofacial reconstruction (**Fig. 2**).

Following 3-dimensional CT imaging, the data are obtained in digital imaging and communications in medicine (DICOM) format and segmented using dedicated

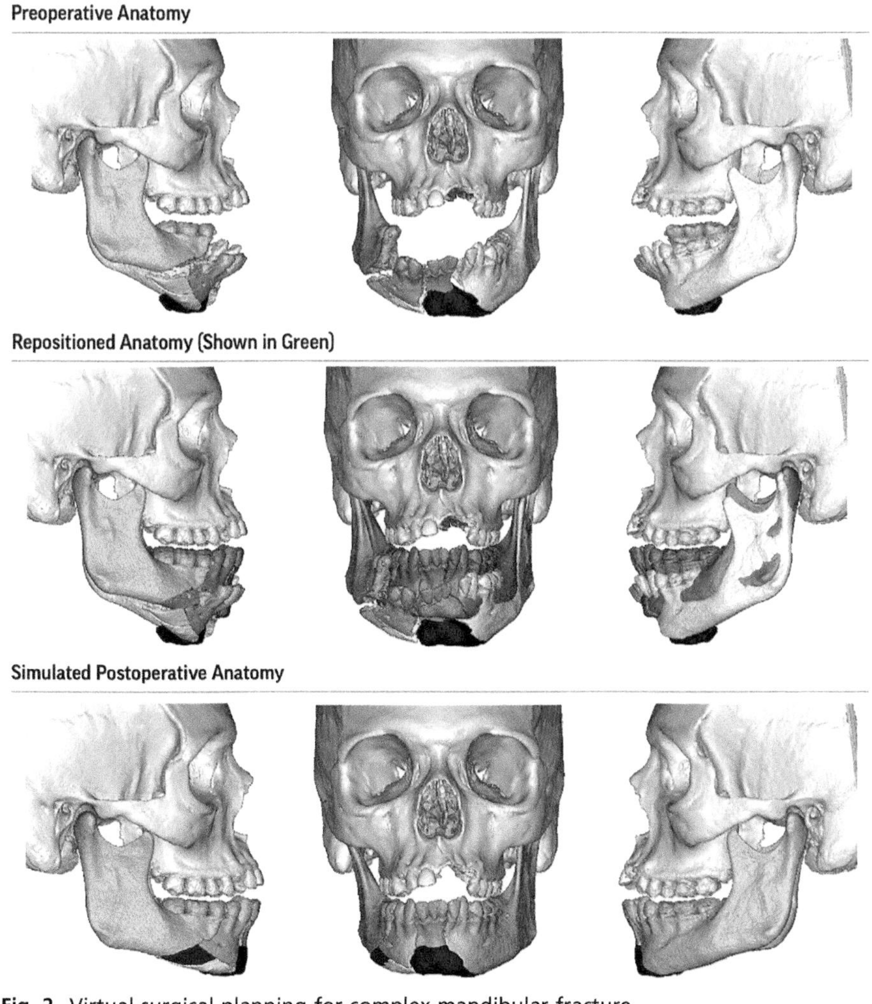

Preoperative Anatomy

Repositioned Anatomy (Shown in Green)

Simulated Postoperative Anatomy

Fig. 2. Virtual surgical planning for complex mandibular fracture.

software (ie, US Food and Drug Administration (FDA)-cleared segmentation and pa-tient data-extraction software). The region of interest is then further segmented from 2-dimensional sections into a 3-dimensional object, either automatically based on software capabilities, or manually following discussion with the surgical team.[6,8] After additional processing, including noise and artifact removal from the images, a 3-dimensional model in the form of stereolithographic (STL) data is extracted. These models can then be loaded onto surgical planning platforms to be used to virtually manipulate bone and soft tissue, reduce fractures, and design osteotomies for more accurate surgical planning (**Fig. 3**).[7,8] In maxillofacial trauma, mirroring is a commonly used technique that involves analyzing the presumably intact, contralateral anatomy to reconstruct the fractured area of interest, especially in cases of orbital reconstruc-tion.[9] The mirrored anatomy can serve as a basis for VSP and patient-specific implant (PSI) design.

VSP is a beneficial tool that can improve the precision and accuracy of implant and hardware placement in maxillofacial reconstruction. VSP can also be used in conjunc-tion with 3-dimensional printing to create models of the defect site and bone segments to practice positioning and fixation, and evaluate aesthetic outcomes.[7]

THREE-DIMENSIONAL PRINTING MODELS

In 1986, Charles Hull introduced to the world US Patent 4,575,330, entitled "Apparatus for Production of Three-Dimensional Objects by Stereolithography." This ingenious design detailed a "stepwise laminar buildup of [a] desired object" from a digital source.

Preoperative Anatomy

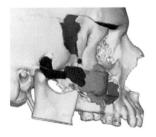 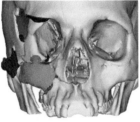 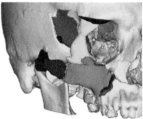

Simulated Postoperative Anatomy

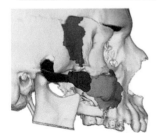 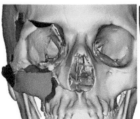 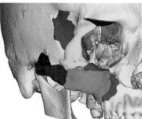

Fig. 3. Virtual surgical planning of a complex midface fracture demonstrating preoperative anatomy and simulated postoperative anatomy.

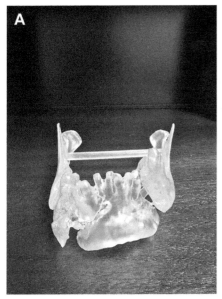 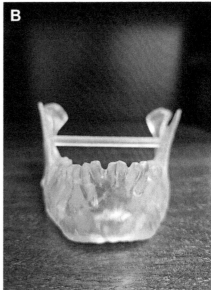

Fig. 4. (*A*) 3-dimensional printed model of a comminuted mandible fracture (*B*) 3-dimensional printed model of simulated post-operative anatomy.

Initially created for application within the manufacturing industry, this technology has over the years been used in many different facets, including personal, military, commercial use, and health care (**Fig. 4**).

There are multiple advantages and disadvantages to the use of computer-aided design (CAD) and computer-aided manufacturing (CAM).[10] Advantages include better cosmetic and functional results in the setting of difficult anatomic locations or defects. On the contrary, however, when arguing against the use of CAD/CAM in reconstruction, many point to the higher cost of methods and materials, its disproportionate reliance on technology, and the necessity to follow a predetermined and rigid surgical plan as disadvantages. The cosmetic is difficult to quantify because of the subjective nature of the matter; however, Padilla's metanalysis did not show any significant flap or hardware-related complications.

Indeed, the cost considerations are real. One study that analyzed the cost comparisons of CAD/CAM versus conventional showed a 4200 Euro increase in the cost of the physical product.[11] This was, however, balanced by money saved in operating room time saved. The study showed that by using precurved plates, approximately 120 minutes of operating room time were saved. With the average per minute cost of operating room time being 35 Euros, the savings showed a 4200 Euro decrease in cost. Using precurved plates had a net-neutral cost, while having the benefit of decreased surgical time, which is shown to be associated with a reduction in hospital days, post-anesthesia care unit (PACU) days, and complications. This cost-saving has been characterized in many other articles.[12]

One way of creating a more sustainable and cost-effective approach to CAD/CAM is by the purchase of one's own 3-dimensional printer and software.[13] The cost of the approach first includes purchasing a printer (typically $500 to $2500). Once this fixed cost is accounted for, raw materials are inexpensive: a human skull 3-dimensional printout may cost about $3.40, and an ear printout costs less than $0.50. A fracture may be contoured before surgery using this method. Note that this method can also allow the surgical trainee to practice manual plate bending and operative planning.

CUTTING AND DRILLING GUIDES

Virtual planning software, used in conjunction with 3-dimensional printing, allows for the development of surgical templates for intraoperative use. These templates are frequently used as cutting guides to aid in the precision of harvesting and positioning pieces of the fibula for accurate mandibular reconstruction.[7] These templates can also be used to ensure adequate resection in mandibular lesions and have been shown to facilitate the preservation of the inferior alveolar nerve.[14] In these situations, cutting guides are useful to visually study the relationship between the mandibular lesion and the inferior alveolar nerve in each patient to facilitate precise cuts, prevent

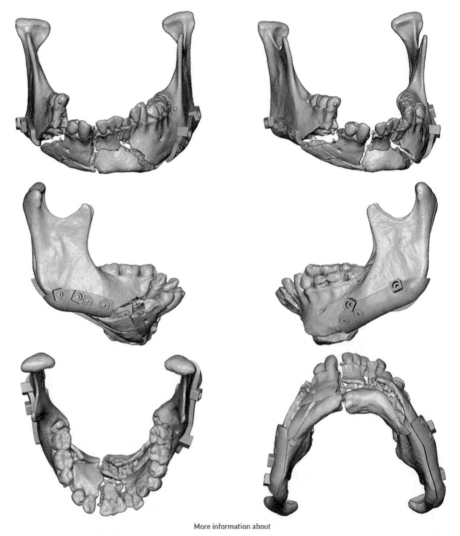

More information about

Fig. 5. Example of drilling guides.

hypoesthesia, and reduce operative time. Similarly, in maxillofacial trauma, surgical templates can serve as drill guides (**Fig. 5**) or cutting guides to facilitate the correct positioning of implants at predetermined depths and angles.[15] Surgical guides, often accurate to the millimeter scale, are printed using sterile, bioinert materials such as acrylonitrile butadiene styrene (ABS), polymethylmethacrylate (PMMA), or polypropylene.

Three-dimensional imaging and printing advances have enabled surgeons to assess different approaches, options, and outcomes in a virtual environment. This virtual surgery planning, together with physical modeling of the defects, custom cutting and positioning guides, and patient-specific implants, has significantly aided the surgeon in his or her approach to complex maxillofacial reconstruction.

PATIENT-SPECIFIC IMPLANTS

Traditional premade implants often require intraoperative adjustments, leading to longer operative time, and they usually offer suboptimal results.[16,17] Advances in 3-dimensional imaging and printing have led to increased utilization of PSIs in repairing complex maxillofacial defects. The ability of some medical companies to provide PSI within 3 to 5 working days can facilitate routine use in the treatment of acute maxillofacial trauma.[18] Several studies support that PSI offers higher accuracy, better site adaptation, and shortened operating time compared with prebent or premade implants that require intraoperative adjustments.[16,19,20]

Implants or grafts traditionally used for these defects have included allografts of bone or cartilage, which often have unpredictable resorption and donor site morbidity rates to an array of alloplastic materials such as titanium, porous polyethylene, and polyetheretherketone (PEEK)[16]

Titanium is a commonly used biocompatible, inert material that allows osseointegration within the underlying bone. Titanium implants remain the material of choice for maxillofacial internal fixation and reconstruction. Titanium reconstruction plates are flat or have a prefabricated bend, and they usually require intraoperative bending. Bending a plate to fit a patient's particular defect can be time-consuming and can also weaken the integrity of the plate.

PEEK is a semicrystalline polyaromatic linear polymer that was developed in 1978 and was initially used in industrial applications (**Fig. 6**).[21] In the 1990s, it emerged as a high-performance, thermoplastic, implantable contender having good biocompatibility and the potential to replace metal implant materials.[6,17,21,22] PEEK has radiographic translucency and does not produce artifacts on imaging, which is an advantage when compared with titanium.[7,21] PEEK is similar to cortical bone in its elasticity and can be trimmed intraoperatively if needed.[22]

Large orbital defects are frequently recognized as a surgical challenge for which patient-specific implants may be useful. Several studies indicate a better outcome in orbital surgery with patient-specific implants when compared with generic manually fabricated or preformed titanium mesh implants.[17,18] However, in times when cost-efficient health care is often emphasized, the decision to pursue a PSI should be made carefully. For example, titanium mesh implants, bent intraoperatively, can be particularly disadvantageous in cases with large or irregular bone defects with secondary changes in orbital volume because of increased risk of implant malposition or insufficient bulk, leading to enophthalmos and diplopia.[17] PSI can offer the advantage of providing additional volume to areas with any fat or soft tissue loss for which a traditional plate cannot compensate. PSI should also be considered in multiple wall

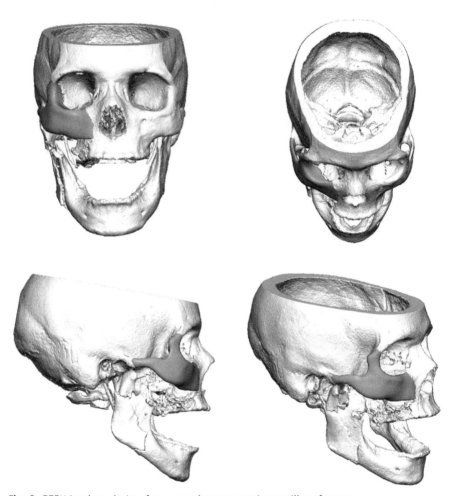

Fig. 6. PEEK implant design for a complex zygomaticomaxillary fracture.

fractures, as they have a higher revision rate with the classical preformed implants when compared with single wall fractures.[18]

In conclusion, PSI may be most useful in revision surgeries, irregular thickness defects, and orbital rims.

INTRAOPERATIVE COMPUTED TOMOGRAPHY

Since Rontgen's discovery of X-rays in 1895, medical imaging had undergone rapid development. First used intraoperatively for fluoroscopy and angiography, these imaging modalities soon became reliable enough to be used even for neurosurgical resections, ensuring that even the smallest residual of disease is excised.[23]

Intraoperative CT has shown remarkable efficacy as an intraoperative tool for the management of chondromyxoid fibroma (CMF) trauma (**Fig. 7**). A retrospective case series from the Legacy Emanuel Medical Center, Head and Neck Institute, in Portland Oregon, analyzed the CT-directed revision rates for different fracture subsites.[24] It was concluded that intraoperative CT usage should not be performed for Le Fort I and

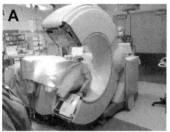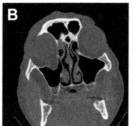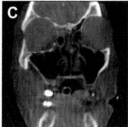

Fig. 7. (A) Portable CT scanner. (B) Preoperative CT showing a right orbital floor defect. (C) Intraoperative CT obtained after reconstruction of the left orbital floor.

frontal sinus fractures because of CT-guided revisions of 8% and 0%. In the author's opinion, the revision rates were high enough to justify the usage for LeFort II/III, zygomaticomaxillary complex fractures, and isolated orbit fractures (**Table 1**).

Similarly, the authors created a protocol to identify elements of zygomaticomaxillary complex (ZMC) fractures that required CT-directed revision. ZMCs that require orbital floor reconstruction, where adjacent fractures require fixation and/or when at least 2 axes are displaced at least 5 mm justified the use of intraoperative CT. Other studies have also shown a statistically significant association between postoperative diplopia and a surgical indication of entrapment/revision and the use of intraoperative CT.[25]

Image-Guided Navigation

The use of image-guided systems (IGS) during surgery has been well-established in the field of endoscopic sinus and skull base surgery.[26] These systems use preoperative CT imaging and are correlated with multiple reference points of the patient's

Table 1
Computed tomography-directed revision rates

Injury Pattern and/or Indication for Scan	Number of Scans	CT-Directed Revision Rate
Isolated orbital fracture	80	31%
Zygomaticomaxillary complex fracture	71	24%
Le Fort II or III fracture	26	23%
Le Fort I fracture	12	8%
Naso-orbital–ethmoidal fracture	13	23%
Mandible fracture	16	13%
Frontal sinus fracture	14	0%
Hardware removal	4	0%
Temporomandibular replacement	2	0%
Craniofacial implant	1	0%
Overall data	212	28%

Data from Cuddy K, Khatib B, Bell RB, et al. Use of intraoperative computed tomography in cranio-maxillofacial trauma surgery. J Oral Maxillofac Surg 2018;76(5):1016-1025.

anatomy via a process of registration at the time of surgery. It provides tracking of instruments in real time on the preoperative imaging.

The use of IGS as an intraoperative tool for the management of complex and revision maxillofacial injuries is an obvious extension of this technology.[27] This provides an option for intraoperative assessment of reduction and hardware position by placing the navigation pointer at the surface of the hardware. It has the benefit over intraoperative CT of not requiring additional radiation exposure to the patient. It also can be used in conjunction with other computer-assisted techniques such as virtual planning and intraoperative CT imaging.

A limited factor for the use of IGS is changes in the soft tissue at the time of surgery from the time of the preoperative imaging, as this can affect the accuracy of the registration.

SUMMARY

The treatment of complex and secondary facial trauma injuries can present a significant challenge for the craniomaxillofacial surgeon. The application of new and upcoming technologies and the application of already existing ones in different ways, provide useful tools for potentially improving outcomes. As seen here, most of the benefits of the use of such technologies come mostly from studies with low-grade evidence. Further research is needed to truly assess the impact of these tools in such patients.

CLINICS CARE POINTS

- High-definition computed tomography (CT) provides improved diagnosis and treatment planning for complex and secondary maxillofacial reconstruction, which can improve surgical outcomes.
- Virtual surgical planning (VSP) is a beneficial tool that can improve the precision and accuracy of implant and hardware placement in maxillofacial reconstruction.
- Patient-specific implants (PSI) should be considered in revision surgeries, irregular thickness defects, and orbital rims.
- The use of intraoperative CT permits real-time revision of adequate reduction and implant placement that improves surgical outcomes.
- The use of image-guided systems (IGS) provides an option for intraoperative assessment of reduction and hardware position without radiation exposure to the patient.

DISCLOSURE

The authors have no conflicts of interest to declare. All coauthors have seen and agree with the contents of the manuscript, and there is no financial interest to report.

REFERENCES

1. Laine FJ, Conway WF, Laskin DM. Radiology of maxillofacial trauma. Curr Probl Diagn Radiol 1993;22(4):145–88.
2. Roth FS, Kokoska MS, Awwad EE, et al. The identification of mandible fractures by helical computed tomography and panorex tomography. J Craniofac Surg 2005;16(3):394–9.

3. Nezafati S, Ghavimi M, Javadrashid R, et al. Comparison of accuracy of computed tomography scan and ultrasonography in the diagnosis of mandibular fractures. Dent Res J 2020;17(3):225–30.
4. Tanrikulu R, Erol B. Comparison of computed tomography with conventional radiography for midfacial fractures. Dentomaxillofac Radiol 2001;30(3):141–6.
5. Fernandes R, DiPasquale J. Computer-aided surgery using 3D rendering of maxillofacial pathology and trauma. Int J Med Robot 2007;3(3):203–6.
6. Herford AS, Miller M, Lauritano F, et al. The use of virtual surgical planning and navigation in the treatment of orbital trauma. Chin J Traumatol 2017;20(1):9–13.
7. Nyberg EL, Farris AL, Hung BP, et al. 3D-printing technologies for craniofacial rehabilitation, reconstruction, and regeneration. Ann Biomed Eng 2017;45(1):45–57.
8. Zoabi A, Redenski I, Oren D, et al. 3D printing and virtual surgical planning in oral and maxillofacial surgery. J Clin Med 2022;11(9):2385.
9. Bly RA, Chang SH, Cudejkova M, et al. Computer-guided orbital reconstruction to improve outcomes. JAMA Facial Plast Surg 2013;15(2):113–20.
10. Padilla PL, Mericli AF, Largo RD, et al. Computer-aided design and manufacturing versus conventional surgical planning for head and neck reconstruction: a systematic review and meta-analysis. Plast Reconstr Surg 2021;148(1):183–92.
11. Rodriguez-Arias JP, Tapia B, Pampin MM, et al. Clinical outcomes and cost analysis of fibula free flaps: a retrospective comparison of CAD/CAM versus conventional technique. J Pers Med 2022;12(6):930.
12. Tarsitano A, Battaglia S, Crimi S, et al. Is a computer-assisted design and computer-assisted manufacturing method for mandibular reconstruction economically viable? J Cranio-Maxillo-Fac Surg 2016;44(7):795–9.
13. Gerstle TL, Ibrahim AMS, Kim PS, et al. A plastic surgery application in evolution: three-dimensional printing. Plast Reconstr Surg 2014;133(2):446–51.
14. De Ketele A, Meeus J, Shaheen E, et al. The usefulness of cutting guides for resection or biopsy of mandibular lesions: a technical note and case report. J Stomatol Oral Maxillofac Surg 2023;124(1):101272.
15. Dings JPJ, Verhamme L, TJJ Maal, et al. Reliability and accuracy of skin-supported surgical templates for computer-planned craniofacial implant placement, a comparison between surgical templates: with and without bony fixation. J Cranio-Maxillo-Fac Surg 2019;47(6):977–83.
16. Alasseri N, Alasraj A. Patient-specific implants for maxillofacial defects: challenges and solutions. Maxillofac Plast Reconstr Surg 2020;42(1):15.
17. Habib LA, Yoon MK. Patient specific implants in orbital reconstruction: a pilot study. Am J Ophthalmol Case Rep 2021;24:101222.
18. Schlittler F, Vig N, Burkhard JP, et al. What are the limitations of the non-patient-specific implant in titanium reconstruction of the orbit? Br J Oral Maxillofac Surg 2020;58(9):e80–5.
19. Baumann A, Sinko K, Dorner G. Late reconstruction of the orbit with patient-specific implants using computer-aided planning and navigation. J Oral Maxillofac Surg 2015;73(12 Suppl):S101–6.
20. Rana M, Chui CH, Wagner M, et al. Increasing the accuracy of orbital reconstruction with selective laser-melted patient-specific implants combined with intraoperative navigation. J Oral Maxillofac Surg 2015;73(6):1113–8.
21. Sarfraz S, Mantynen PH, Laurila M, et al. Comparison of titanium and PEEK medical plastic implant materials for their bacterial biofilm formation properties. Polymers 2022;14(18):3862.

22. Jarvinen S, Suojanen J, Kormi E, et al. The use of patient specific polyetherether-ketone implants for reconstruction of maxillofacial deformities. J Cranio-Maxillo-Fac Surg 2019;47(7):1072–6.
23. Nimsky C, Carl B. Historical, current, and future intraoperative imaging modal-ities. Neurosurg Clin N Am 2017;28(4):453–64.
24. Cuddy K, Khatib B, Bell RB, et al. Use of intraoperative computed tomography in craniomaxillofacial trauma surgery. J Oral Maxillofac Surg 2018;76(5):1016–25.
25. Causbie J, Walters B, Lally J, et al. Complications Following Orbital Floor Repair: Impact of Intraoperative Computed Tomography Scan and Implant Material. Facial Plast Surg Aesthet Med 2020;22(5):315–400.
26. Schmale IL, Vandelaar LJ, Luong AU, et al. Image-guided surgery and intraoper-ative imaging in rhinology: clinical update and current state of the art. Ear Nose Throat J 2021;100(10):NP475–86.
27. Nijmeh AD, Goodger NM, Hawkes D, et al. Image-guided navigation in oral and maxillofacial surgery. Br J Oral Maxillofac Surg 2005;43(4):294–302.

Complications of Mandibular Fracture Repair

Anna Celeste Gibson, MD*, Tyler Branch Merrill, MD,
Jennings Russell Boyette, MD

KEYWORDS

- Mandibular fracture complications • Mandible fracture complication management
- Mandibular fracture repair • Postoperative care
- Temporomandibular joint (TMJ) ankylosis

KEY POINTS

- Published mandibular fracture repair complication rates can range from single digits to more than 50%.
- The most common mandibular fracture complications include infection, hardware failure, nonunion, malocclusion, dental-related complications, temporal joint ankylosis, nerve injury, and pediatric-specific complications.
- Appropriate preoperative considerations, intraoperative technique, and meticulous postoperative care can reduce the rates of complications.

Abbreviations	
ORIF	open Reduction Internal Fixation
MMF	maxillomandibular Fixation
IMF	intermaxillary Fixation

INTRODUCTION

Mandible fracture management has evolved dramatically from an era of reliance on maxillomandibular fixation (MMF) and splinting to the present day where many fractures can be approached intraorally and internally fixated. Improvements in imaging have allowed for more precise diagnosis and clear surgical planning while improvements in instrumentation and plating systems have allowed for improved surgical access and more reliable outcomes. Therefore, the variety of surgical complications associated with mandibular fractures, and their incidences, has continued to change

Department of Otolaryngology–Head and Neck Surgery, University of Arkansas for Medical Sciences, 4301 West Markham Street, Slot #543, Little Rock, AR 72205, USA
* Corresponding author.
E-mail address: acgibson@uams.edu

Otolaryngol Clin N Am 56 (2023) 1137–1150
https://doi.org/10.1016/j.otc.2023.05.008
0030-6665/23/Published by Elsevier Inc.

as well. Although some complications may be minor and only require a period of supportive care, others can be quite devastating to patients and require significant intervention. The overall scope of complications related to fracture repair is challenging to appraise because there are varying fracture types, fixation strategies, degrees of surgeon expertise, and patient comorbidities. That may explain why published overall complication rates can range from single digits to more than 50%, with many of these sources based on small case series, and some from decades past.[1–4] For this reason, it is necessary to parse out and compartmentalize these complications in order to begin to infer their causes and how they can be avoided. This article aims to assess the most common and most concerning complications that can occur secondary to management of mandibular fractures by examining categories of complication types.

Infection

- *The routine use of preoperative antibiotics does not prevent infectious complications. However, perioperative antibiotics are recommended.*
- *Delaying surgical repair does not lead to increased infection rates.*

Infection rates are widely variable in mandibular fracture repair likely due to the differing definitions. Certain factors do portend higher rates of infection. Patient-specific factors such as tobacco use, substance use, comorbidities, and poor oral hygiene have been found to have a significant association with infection rates.[5–8] Fracture-specific factors such as number of mandibular fractures sustained and number of treated fractures have a significant correlation with infection. Surgery-dependent factors also contribute to higher rates. Internal fixation of fractures has been found to have higher rates of infection than external fixation. A combination of the two approaches has been found to have the highest rate.[5]

Historically, it was thought that a mandibular angle fracture with the third molar in line of the fracture increased the risk of infection, and therefore, some providers extracted the tooth regardless of its viability. A meta-analysis by Bobrowski and colleagues found no significant difference in infection rates with removal or retention of the third molar in the fracture line.[9] Another debated topic is the association of time to treatment and infection rate. It has been found that the delay of treatment by several days does not increase the risk of infection or other complications.[10,11]

The utility of antibiotics with mandible fracture repair is debated. Before the Centers for Medicare and Medicaid Services established a mandate of intraoperative antibiotic prophylaxis, it was already a commonplace practice.[12] The use of short-term perioperative antibiotics is still substantiated in the literature to reduce infection.[13] Variation exists with the use of preoperative and postoperative antibiotics. A national database study from 2021 found that the use of preoperative antibiotics (prescribed within 10 days before repair) did not improve mandibular repair outcomes.[14] Other studies have similarly found no infectious risk reduction with the use of postoperative antibiotics.[6] Some surgeons will still advocate for the use of preoperative antibiotics in cases of open fractures or those fractures involving an injured tooth; however, the routine use of preoperative antibiotics is not recommended.[14,15]

To manage active infection, it is recommended to explore the wound and perform thorough washout. If hardware failure is present, the hardware should be removed and the mandible should be fixated with more rigid hardware.[1]

Hardware-Related Complications

- *Wound dehiscence and hardware exposure is more common in smokers.*
- *Removal of exposed or loose hardware can be delayed until bony union occurs.*

Although hardware failure can have differing definitions in the literature, it is generally thought of as loose screws, loose plates, and/or dehiscence and exposure of the hardware. True fracturing of plates is rare; therefore, either hardware exposure or extrusion is a better term to describe the clinical scenario. Hardware problems can occur simultaneously or because of other mandibular fracture complications. A study by Gutta and colleagues reported the need for failed hardware removal to be 15.4% with 10% of those cases presenting with infection.[4] Hardware complications can also present with wound dehiscence. In the case of wound dehiscence, the hardware does not necessarily need to be removed immediately. One study reviewed wound dehiscence in 69 fractures of healthy patients who were nonsmokers and nonalcohol users. In this study, the authors managed dehiscence conservatively by using irrigation with warm saline and chlorhexidine mouthwash and had success with secondary healing.[16] However, some argue that wound dehiscence will likely lead to eventual hardware removal overtime, therefore, one might consider hardware removal once bone healing is confirmed.

In theory, some have questioned the utility of resorbable plates to reduce complications such has hardware failure and need for removal. One systematic review and meta-analysis found that the use of resorbable versus metallic implants had no significant difference in outcomes for patients.[17]

Nonunion

- *Nonunion is likely the result of inadequate fixation.*
- *Concomitant infection does not preclude revision internal, rigid fixation.*

Nonunion across the fracture site is less of a distinct complication than the result or culmination of some of the other complications such as infection, inadequate fixation, or hardware failure. The incidence of nonunion has remained relatively stable (<4%) despite the advent of new techniques of mandibular repair.[18,19] However, the use of sturdy titanium plates and rigid load-bearing techniques do make motion at the fracture line less likely.[20] Certain factors associated with higher rates of nonunion include multiple fractures, fractures of the mandibular body and fractures in edentulous patients; these factors intuitively decrease the stability of the repair and have a compromised blood supply, which can lead to poor healing.[19,21]

Patient-related factors may also have some impact on bone healing. Drug abuse and tobacco smoking are associated with increased complication rates in general.[22–24] Age does not appear to be factor, except in cases of the atrophic mandible.[23,25] In theory, patient compliance is thought to affect the stability of fracture repair and can lead to nonunion. Earlier studies have shown that patient noncompliance is quite high within this patient population; however, these studies have reported that noncomplicance seems to have little impact on increasing complications such as nonunion.[26,27] Postoperative diet restriction to a no-chew diet for up to 6 weeks is commonly recommended in order to allow for stability of fractures and prevention of nonunion; noncompliance with this instruction is often identified as the inciting factor for nonunion. However, in a prospective study of 375 patients, there was no significant increase in complications with a gradual return to regular diet at 2 or 4 weeks compared with 6 weeks postoperatively.[28]

It is suspected that many cases of nonunion are the result of inadequate fixation by the surgeon. However, this is challenging to assess in the published literature because most studies are retrospective outcomes studies that do not specifically report the degree of fixation or fixation strategy for individual fracture sites. Cases of nonunion due to inadequate fixation will often present with signs and symptoms of infection or loosening hardware and therefore, upon analysis, these problems may be attributed as the cause of poor bone healing. Therefore, initial fracture characteristics, such as comminution, should be considered when selecting a fixation strategy between load-sharing techniques and load-bearing techniques.

The relationship between infection and nonunion is cyclic and important to understand. Infection stimulates fibroblastic activity over osteoclastic/osteoblastic proliferation and leads to more fibrous than osseous development.[29] Mobility across the fracture is thought to reduce revascularization of the bone and may lead to an increased risk of infection of the devitalized bone.[30] Therefore, in terms of nonunion, antibiotic treatment alone is insufficient to treat the infection or poor bone healing. Instead, stability must be reestablished. That can be restored with rigid, load-bearing fixation, and removal of any loose hardware or devitalized bone and dentition (**Figs. 1 and 2**). Many surgeons and infectious disease specialists are uncomfortable with the notion of implanting new titanium plates into an infected surgical site but the interplay between mobility and infection must be recognized to fully treat both problems. Studies demonstrating successful treatment of infected mandibular nonunion with rigid internal fixation are well documented.[31,32] With this management, the use of external fixator systems can also be avoided.

Malocclusion

- Malocclusion is the consequence of malreduction and, if severe, should be revised quickly.

A primary goal of treatment of mandibular fractures in restoration of preinjury bite. Malocclusion noted early in recovery likely indicates poor reduction during surgery. The true incidence of malocclusion after surgery is difficult to determine because this complication is not reported in almost all retrospective studies. In the early postoperative period, some patients will have muscle swelling and trismus, and subtle occlusal changes can be noticed. However, a true malreduction resulting in malocclusion is typically quite obvious. Consideration of swift revision before malunion should be strongly considered. If MMF was performed, loosening wires or removing elastics to allow for manipulation in pursuit of restoration of occlusion could also be considered.[33,34] If malocclusion becomes apparent in late recovery, one can consider both surgical and nonsurgical treatment options. In terms of surgical treatments, a variety

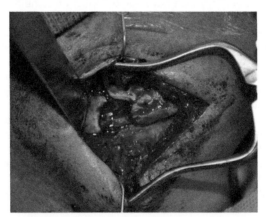

Fig. 1. Nonunion of a right mandibular body fracture. Patient complained of segment mobility with intermittent purulent drainage from a submandibular skin wound. Miniplates were removed and bony sequestrum was debrided.

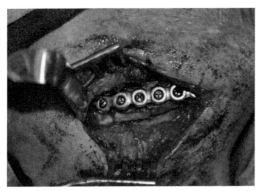

Fig. 2. Iliac crest bone graft placed into defect with a load-bearing reconstruction plate. Cancellous bone grafts later packed into any remaining space between segments.

of orthognathic procedures can be considered based on the nature of the malocclusion. In less severe cases, nonsurgical treatments can include orthodontic treatment, prosthodontic treatment or splint therapy.[35]

Dental Complications

- *Removal of uninjured teeth involved in a fracture does not decrease complications but may aid in the reduction of the fracture segments.*

The management of teeth within the fracture lines has been long debated. As previously mentioned, some providers have opted to extract any teeth within the line of fracture due to concern that it would act as a nidus of infection. One article by Chrcanovic included 27 studies in their analysis of teeth within the fracture site. They recommended to not remove or reposition tooth buds unless they show signs of infection. Similarly, they recommend to not remove intact teeth if they show no evidence of severe loosening or inflammatory change. Their recommendation was to follow-up teeth within fracture lines radiographically for one year.[36] However, dental extraction is recommended by many surgeons when the tooth in the line of the fracture restricts accurate reduction of the fracture.[24,30]

Tooth root injury is a concern when inserting screws into the mandible both with internal fixation and with intermaxillary fixation (IMF) screws. If a tooth root is injured, outcomes can range from no impact on tooth health to need for endodontic treatment or even tooth loss. Multiple studies evaluating screw placement in the adult population have found the rate of tooth root injury to be up to 17%.[37] Thankfully, in these studies, long-term sequelae were much less common.[38–40] Among the studies, tooth root injury appeared to be more common with IMF screws as opposed to screws securing plates to the bone. If tooth root damage is suspected, it has been recommended to follow the patient for at least 4 to 6 months with imaging as needed based on symptoms with a low threshold for referral for endodontic treatment.[41]

Nerve Injury

- *Facial nerve injury is a rare complication of condylar fracture approaches. Endoscopic condylar fracture repair puts the nerve at less risk.*
- *Sensory nerve injury is a common complication and can be avoided with good surgical technique. If nerve recovery has not occurred after 3 months, nerve grafting repair can be considered.*

Both motor and sensory nerves can be injured during surgical repair of mandibular fractures. Facial nerve injury secondary to repair of mandibular fractures predominantly occurs during open treatment of condylar fractures. A systematic review and meta-analysis published in 2017 by Al-Moraissi and colleagues evaluated the rates of various approaches to the condyle.[42] This study analyzed 96 studies and included 3873 patients. For the intraoral approach, the study differentiated between patients treated with and without transbuccal instrumentation as well as the endoscopic-assisted technique. The intraoral approach without transbuccal instrumentation was found to be the safest with respect to the facial nerve with a transient paresis rate under 1% and no cases of permanent facial nerve paralysis. With transbuccal instrumentation, the transient paresis rate went up to 2.7%. Still no permanent paralysis was seen. The endoscopic-assisted approach was seen to have a slightly higher rate of transient paresis (4.2%) again with no permanent paralysis.

The submandibular approach to the mandible can put the marginal mandibular nerve at risk. As the nerve exits the parotid, it runs deep to the platysma and the investing fascia. Its course is somewhat variable in its relationship to the mandible because it crosses the facial vessels.[43] It follows that the marginal mandibular branch, in particular, is at risk during the submandibular approach. Al-Moraissi and colleagues found that the rate of transient injury in studies using a traditional low submandibular approach (Risdon approach) to be much higher at 15.3%. The permanent paralysis rate was 2.2%. Contrary to this, patients treated with the high submandibular approach had no examples of transient paresis (0%), and only one patient (0.61%) with permanent paralysis.

The retromandibular approach with retroparotid dissection had a transient paresis rate of 19% and permanent paralysis rate of 1.5% while the retromandibular approach with transparotid dissection had a transient rate of 14.4% and permanent rate of 1.4%. The retromandibular preparotid transmasseteric approach had a lower rate of paresis with a transient rate between 2.3% and 3.4%. No examples of permanent paresis were seen with this technique.

Preauricular approaches were separated into three categories: transparotid dissection, deep subfascial dissection, and a traditional preauricular approach with subfascial dissection. The preauricular transparotid showed a transient paresis rate of 2.8% with no cases of permanent paresis. Deep subfascial dissection was not commonly used but no cases of transient or permanent facial nerve injury were found. The traditional preauricular approach with subfascial dissection resulted in a transient paresis rate of 10% and a permanent rate of 0.3%. The retroauricular approach had a transient paresis rate of 3% and a permanent paralysis rate of 0%.

In terms of sensory nerve injury, internal fixation has been shown to have higher rates of sensory nerve injury than closed treatment.[44] This has been found to be higher in patients with significant displacement (>5 mm), patients with normal preoperative function and in cases involving operator experience under 3 years.[45] However, in patients with traumatic, preoperative, neurosensory deficit, early treatment can reduce time to recovery.[46] Although intraoral approaches may offer an improved cosmesis and reduced risk of facial nerve injury, they can result in risk to the inferior alveolar nerve and mental nerve. Parasymphyseal fractures especially can put the mental nerve at risk because they require skeletonization of the nerve for exposure of the inferior aspect of the fracture. Another common instance of inferior alveolar nerve injury is placement of a bicortical screw into the mandibular canal. Preoperative and intraoperative review of radiographs can aid in identifying and avoiding the course of the nerve during screw placement. A prospective study assessed the subjective and objective recovery of neurologic function after intraoral repair of mandibular fractures. In this study, after 57 days, all patients had recovered sensory function to a two-point discrimination between 2 and 6 mm. It took up to 90 days for all to recover subjective sensation.[47]

In cases of peripheral nerve injury, microsurgical repair can be considered. Bagheri and colleagues described a success rate of 81%.[48] This was echoed by a systematic review, which again found ~80% success rate for repair of peripheral mandibular nerve injuries.[49] Treatments other than neurorrhaphy and nerve grafting have been described have included the following: neurolysis to remove scar tissue impinging the nerve, laser treatment of partial sensory loss, antiepileptics, antidepressants, analgesics, and counseling.[50]

Temporomandibular Joint Ankylosis

- Ankylosis may occur with prolonged joint immobilization and is more common with condylar fractures.
- Attempts to restore normal anatomy with internal fixation and avoid prolonged MMF can help to prevent ankylosis.

Temporomandibular joint (TMJ) ankylosis is a rare sequela of trauma and has most often been linked to condylar fractures.[51] Different authors have found the incidence of ankylosis in condylar fractures to be between 0.4% and 5%.[52–54] Ankylosis classically has been classified as fibrous or bony. Symptoms range from mild progressively worsening jaw movement to complete joint fixation, orofacial deformity (especially in the pediatric population), and pain. It is generally thought that an intra-articular hematoma forms and subsequent fibrosis drives ankylosis.[55]

Although significant research has been done to improve outcomes regarding TMJ ankylosis, it remains a challenging clinical entity with varying management strategies.[56] Although MMF may seem to be an attractive treatment option for patients with condylar fractures, there is concern that immobilization could increase the risk of ankylosis.[57] Avoidance of MMF by internally fixating condylar neck fractures is debated. No gold standard exists at this time, although, it is generally accepted that in cases of significant displacement, joint dislocation, significantly restricted mobility or malocclusion, open reduction, internal fixation (ORIF) should be considered

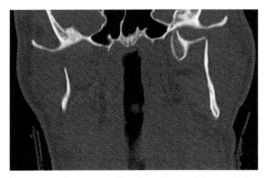

Fig. 3. Maxillofacial computed tomography showing a left condylar neck fracture. The condylar head is dislocated out of the glenoid fossa. The condylar segment is displaced medially. Closed reduction with maxillomandibular fixation would not correct the dislocation and is likely to result in complications such of malocclusion, long-term temporomandibular dysfunction, and possibly joint ankylosis. Recognizing when internal fixation is needed for condylar fractures is key to preventing complications.

(Fig. 3). Schneider and colleagues performed a randomized prospective study comparing ORIF to MMF and found that for fractures of the condylar base, neck and head, ORIF provided improved outcomes both objectively and subjectively when compared with MMF. A recent meta-analysis supported the role of ORIF except in cases of minimally displaced condylar fractures.[58] Another meta-analysis including 859 patients proposed a more nuanced opinion showing that ORIF improved mouth opening but showed no difference between ORIF and MMF in terms of subjective mandibular range-of-motion.[59] It should be noted that in general, subcondylar fractures have a significantly lower rate of ankylosis because the joint capsule remains intact.[60,61] Due to this fact, MMF can be used for a longer period than it should for condylar head fractures.[60]

Fractures of the condylar head (intracapsular/diacapitular) are more prone to ankylosis.[53] These fractures are common and have long been treated with MMF to restore occlusal relationships, although immobilization may predispose the patient to ankylosis. An important consideration is the TMJ disc.[62] A study looking at 51 patients with post-traumatic ankylosis found that all had an intracapsular component.[63] All of these had some sort of disc displacement as well. Therefore, some surgeons have begun to explore ORIF for condylar head fractures in order to restore normal joint anatomy, and initial results are promising in select cases.[64,65]

Once diagnosed, treatment of ankylosis is targeted at correcting any facial deformity, restoring function and mobility of the joint, and preventing progression or reankylosis. Treatment options are variable and no clear consensus has been reached for management. Surgical options generally considered include simple resection, gap arthroplasty, interpositional arthroplasty, autogenous TMJ reconstruction, and alloplastic TMJ reconstruction.[66,67] Choice of surgical offering depends greatly on surgeon's ability and experience. Whatever treatment is pursued, mouth-opening exercises remain a necessary part of recovery. Unfortunately, outcomes are variable, and re-ankylosis is not uncommon.[61]

Pediatric Mandibular Fracture Complications

- *Conservative, closed treatment is preferred if there is good alignment of fracture segments.*
- *Internal fixation plating must be modified in order to avoid screw placement into unerupted dentition.*
- *Closed treatment should be considered for condylar fractures to avoid growth disturbances.*

Pediatric mandibular fractures are less common than adult fractures and complications are much less common.[5] However, there are a few special considerations to keep in mind such as continued growth of the mandible, dentition status, and unerupted teeth. These factors along with the high proportion of incomplete fractures and high osteogenic properties of pediatric bone often sway the decision-making toward conservative therapy in the pediatric population.[67] When pursuing open treatment, a few specific factors are worth consideration: condylar fractures can disrupt growth in a way that results in long-lasting asymmetry, tooth buds can be affected depending on the dentition status of the patient, and the growing mandible may necessitate the removal of titanium plates.

Condyle fractures pose a unique risk to the pediatric population as the condylar neck area drives vertical growth of the ramus.[68] This makes long-term asymmetry a concern when addressing these fractures in children. Although some authors caution about high rates of facial asymmetry,[68,69] a more recent study found much lower rates of facial asymmetry in patients who underwent ORIF for condylar fractures.[70] Patients suffering from asymmetry secondary to mandibular fractures may require orthognathic surgery in the future.[69,71] Although the potential risk is significant, further studies are needed to better define this risk.

Although the presence of tooth buds prompts concern about damaging unerupted teeth, careful technique seems to make this a rare occurrence.[72] Screws should be placed as low as possible on the mandible to avoid the unerupted teeth. A recent retrospective study showed no instances of dental injury in a group of 91 pediatric patients undergoing ORIF for fractures involving the dentate mandible.[73] A systematic review by Bobrowski and colleagues supported this with no tooth bud injury as well.[67] Understanding the anatomical changes that occur at various ages is important in designing a treatment plan.

Bioresorbable plates have been considered for decades in the treatment of pediatric craniomaxillofacial fractures.[74] As the mandible is still growing, the rigidity of metallic plates often necessitates removal in the pediatric patient. Resorbable plates attempt to obviate a second surgery. Advances have made bioresorbable systems stronger and more biocompatible. Three recent systematic reviews resulted in different conclusions. One group found that resorbable plates compared favorably to titanium plates in multiple ways such as overall complication rates, malocclusion rates, reoperation, and infection.[75] However, a later published meta-analysis by a group led by the same author found no significant difference between resorbable plates and titanium plates.[17] Most recently, Pontell and colleagues found no difference other than titanium plates were more likely to require surgical removal.[76] These apparent contradictions show that the relative rarity of ORIF of the mandible in the pediatric population limits the generalizability of data because most of the work of these reviews is derived from retrospective case series.

SUMMARY

Although techniques have improved during the past few decades, complications still can occur when repairing mandibular fractures. Although appropriate preoperative considerations, intraoperative technique, and meticulous postoperative care can reduce the rates of complications, understanding the management of possible complications is imperative for any surgeon undertaking the care of mandibular trauma.

CLINICS CARE POINTS

- The most common mandibular fracture complications include infection, hardware failure, nonunion, malocclusion, dental-related complications, temporal joint ankylosis, nerve injury, and pediatric-specific complications.

- Many complications of mandible fractures occur concurrently or as a result of another complication.

- Patient-related factors such as drug use, tobacco smoking, comorbidities, and poor oral hygiene are associated with increased complication rates.

- Perioperative antibiotic prophylaxis for mandibular fractures is substantiated in the literature to reduce infection.

- Delaying the treatment of mandibular fractures by several days does not increase the risk of infection or other complications.

- There is no consensus on the benefit of resorbable plates over titanium plates regarding hardware failure or pediatric-related complications.

- Malocculsion and nonunion can be the result of malreduction and poor fixation at the time of surgery.
- In theory, postoperative diet restriction to a no-chew diet for up to 6 weeks allows for stability of the fractures and prevention of nonunion; however, there are data that reports diet restriction has little impact on complication rates.
- Studies demonstrating successful treatment of infected mandibular nonunion with rigid internal fixation are well documented.
- Teeth within the fracture line does not necessitate removal; however, one might consider extraction if the tooth prevents adequate reduction.
- Intraoral approaches may offer reduced risk of facial nerve injury, however, can result in increased risk to the inferior alveolar nerve and mental nerve.

CONFLICTS OF INTEREST AND SOURCES OF FUNDING

None declared.

REFERENCES

1. Pickrell BB, Hollier LH Jr. Evidence-Based Medicine: Mandible Fractures. Plast Reconstr Surg 2017;140(1):192e–200e.
2. Stacey DH, Doyle JF, Mount DL, et al. Management of mandible fractures. Plast Reconstr Surg 2006;117(3):48e–60e.
3. Passeri LA, Ellis E 3rd, Sinn DP. Complications of nonrigid fixation of mandibular angle fractures. J Oral Maxillofac Surg 1993;51(4):382–4.
4. Gutta R, Tracy K, Johnson C, et al. Outcomes of mandible fracture treatment at an academic tertiary hospital: a 5-year analysis. J Oral Maxillofac Surg 2014;72(3):550–8.
5. Odom EB, Snyder-Warwick AK. Mandible Fracture Complications and Infection: The Influence of Demographics and Modifiable Factors. Plast Reconstr Surg 2016;138(2):282e–9e.
6. Domingo F, Dale E, Gao C, et al. A single-center retrospective review of postoperative infectious complications in the surgical management of mandibular fractures: Postoperative antibiotics add no benefit. J Trauma Acute Care Surg 2016;81(6):1109–14.
7. Furr AM, Schweinfurth JM, May WL. Factors associated with long-term complications after repair of mandibular fractures. Laryngoscope 2006;116(3):427–30.
8. Janaphan K, Hashem I, Smith C, et al. Periodontal disease as a primary cause of surgical site infection in fractures of the mandible: is smoking a confounding variable? Br J Oral Maxillofac Surg 2022;60(10):1424–9.
9. Bobrowski AN, Sonego CL, Chagas Junior OL. Postoperative infection associated with mandibular angle fracture treatment in the presence of teeth on the fracture line: a systematic review and meta-analysis. Int J Oral Maxillofac Surg 2013;42(9):1041–8.
10. Czerwinski M, Parker WL, Correa JA, et al. Effect of treatment delay on mandibular fracture infection rate. Plast Reconstr Surg 2008;122(3):881–5.
11. Lee UK, Rojhani A, Herford AS, et al. Immediate Versus Delayed Treatment of Mandibular Fractures: A Stratified Analysis of Complications. J Oral Maxillofac Surg 2016;74(6):1186–96.

12. SCIP-Inf 1-10: prophylactic antibiotic received within one hour prior to surgical incision. In: Specifications Manual for National Hospital Inpatient Quality Measures. The Joint Commission website, 2010. Accessed March 2023.
13. Andreasen JO, Jensen SS, Schwartz O, et al. A systematic review of prophylactic antibiotics in the surgical treatment of maxillofacial fractures. J Oral Maxillofac Surg 2006;64(11):1664-8.
14. Wick EH, Deutsch B, Kallogjeri D, et al. Effectiveness of Prophylactic Preoperative Antibiotics in Mandible Fracture Repair: A National Database Study. Otolaryngol Head Neck Surg 2021;165(6):798-808.
15. Dawoud BES, Kent S, Henry A, et al. Use of antibiotics in traumatic mandibular fractures: a systematic review and meta-analysis. Br J Oral Maxillofac Surg 2021;59(10):1140-7.
16. Elsayed SA, Abdullah AAB, Dar-Odeh N, et al. Intraoral Wound Dehiscence After Open Reduction Internal Fixation of Mandibular Fractures: A Retrospective Cohort Study. Wounds 2021;33(3):60-4.
17. Chocron Y, Azzi AJ, Cugno S. Resorbable Implants for Mandibular Fracture Fixation: A Systematic Review and Meta-Analysis. Plast Reconstr Surg Glob Open 2019;7(8):e2384.
18. Mathog RH, Boies LR Jr. Nonunion of the mandible. Laryngoscope 1976;86(7): 908-20.
19. Mathog RH, Toma V, Clayman L, et al. Nonunion of the mandible: an analysis of contributing factors. J Oral Maxillofac Surg 2000;58(7):746-53.
20. De Souza M, Oeltjen JC, Panthaki ZJ, et al. Posttraumatic mandibular deformities. J Craniofac Surg 2007;18(4):912-6.
21. Haug RH, Schwimmer A. Fibrous union of the mandible: a review of 27 patients. J Oral Maxillofac Surg 1994;52(8):832-9.
22. Passeri LA, Ellis E 3rd, Sinn DP. Relationship of substance abuse to complications with mandibular fractures. J Oral Maxillofac Surg 1993;51(1):22-5.
23. Gordon PE, Lawler ME, Kaban LB, et al. Mandibular fracture severity and patient health status are associated with postoperative inflammatory complications. J Oral Maxillofac Surg 2011;69(8):2191-7.
24. Hsieh TY, Funamura JL, Dedhia R, et al. Risk Factors Associated With Complications After Treatment of Mandible Fractures. JAMA Facial Plast Surg 2019;21(3): 213-20.
25. Gerbino G, Roccia F, De Gioanni PP, et al. Maxillofacial trauma in the elderly. J Oral Maxillofac Surg 1999;57(7):777-83.
26. Hurrell MJL, David MC, Batstone MD. Patient compliance and mandible fractures: a prospective study. Int J Oral Maxillofac Surg 2019;48(6):759-68.
27. Radabaugh JP, Horn AV, Chan SA, et al. Patient compliance following isolated mandibular fracture repair. Laryngoscope 2017;127(10):2230-5.
28. Manzie T, David MC, Bobinskas A. Return to normal diet following mandibular fractures - how long is long enough? Br J Oral Maxillofac Surg 2021;59(9): 1050-5.
29. Mathog RH. Nonunion of the mandible. Otolaryngol Clin North Am 1983;16(3): 533-47.
30. Perez D, Ellis E 3rd. Complications of Mandibular Fracture Repair and Secondary Reconstruction. Semin Plast Surg 2020;34(4):225-31.
31. Alpert B, Kushner GM, Tiwana PS. Contemporary management of infected mandibular fractures. Craniomaxillofac Trauma Reconstr 2008;1(1):25-9.
32. Mehra P, Van Heukelom E, Cottrell DA. Rigid internal fixation of infected mandibular fractures. J Oral Maxillofac Surg 2009;67(5):1046-51.

33. Kim SY, Choi YH, Kim YK. Postoperative malocclusion after maxillofacial fracture management: a retrospective case study. Maxillofac Plast Reconstr Surg 2018; 40(1):27.

34. Miles BA, Smith JE. Mandibular Fractures. In: Johnson JT, Rosen CA, editors. Bailey's head and neck surgery. 5th edition. Pennsylvania, PA: Lippincott Williams & Wilkins; 2014. p. 1195–208.

35. Khalaf K, Kheder W, El-Kishawi M, et al. The role of prosthetic, orthodontic and implant-supported rehabilitation in the management of secondary malocclusion to maxillofacial trauma- A systematic review. Saudi Dent J 2021;33(4):177–83.

36. Chrcanovic BR. Teeth in the line of mandibular fractures. Oral Maxillofac Surg 2014;18(1):7–24.

37. Schulte-Geers M, Kater W, Seeberger R. Root trauma and tooth loss through the application of pre-drilled transgingival fixation screws. J Cranio-Maxillo-Fac Surg 2012;40(7):e214–7.

38. Borah GL, Ashmead D. The fate of teeth transfixed by osteosynthesis screws. Plast Reconstr Surg 1996;97(4):726–9.

39. Balaji P, Balaji SM. Open reduction and internal fixation: Screw injury - Retrospective study. Indian J Dent Res 2017;28(3):304–8.

40. Hartwig S, Boettner A, Doll C, et al. Drill-related root injury caused by intraoperative intermaxillary fixation: an analysis of 1067 screw applications. Dent Traumatol 2017;33(1):45–50.

41. Cornelius CP, Ehrenfeld M. The Use of MMF Screws: Surgical Technique, Indications, Contraindications, and Common Problems in Review of the Literature. Craniomaxillofac Trauma Reconstr 2010;3(2):55–80.

42. Al-Moraissi EA, Louvrier A, Colletti G, et al. Does the surgical approach for treating mandibular condylar fractures affect the rate of seventh cranial nerve injuries? A systematic review and meta-analysis based on a new classification for surgical approaches. J Cranio-Maxillo-Fac Surg 2018;46(3):398–412.

43. Balagopal PG, George NA, Sebastian P. Anatomic variations of the marginal mandibular nerve. Indian J Surg Oncol 2012;3(1):8–11.

44. Halpern LR, Kaban LB, Dodson TB. Perioperative neurosensory changes associated with treatment of mandibular fractures. J Oral Maxillofac Surg 2004;62(5): 576–81.

45. Song Q, Li S, Patil PM. Inferior alveolar and mental nerve injuries associated with open reduction and internal fixation of mandibular fractures: a Seven Year retrospective study. J Cranio-Maxillo-Fac Surg 2014;42(7):1378–81.

46. Tabrizi R, Pourdanesh F, Khoshnik PL, et al. Does the Lag Time Between Injury and Treatment Play a Role in Recovery of Inferior Alveolar Nerve Neurosensory Disturbances Following Mandibular Body Fracture? J Craniofac Surg 2019; 30(7):2128–30.

47. Cillo JE Jr, Godwin S, Becker E, et al. Neurosensory Recovery Following Mental Nerve Skeletonization in Intraoral Open Reduction and Internal Fixation of Mandible Fractures. J Oral Maxillofac Surg 2021;79(1):183–91.

48. Bagheri SC, Meyer RA, Cho SH, et al. Microsurgical repair of the inferior alveolar nerve: success rate and factors that adversely affect outcome. J Oral Maxillofac Surg 2012;70(8):1978–90.

49. Weyh A, Pucci R, Valentini V, et al. Injuries of the Peripheral Mandibular Nerve, Evaluation of Interventions and Outcomes: A Systematic Review. Craniomaxillofac Trauma Reconstr 2021;14(4):337–48.

50. Coulthard P, Kushnerev E, Yates JM, et al. Interventions for iatrogenic inferior alveolar and lingual nerve injury. Cochrane Database Syst Rev 2014;4: CD005293.
51. Movahed R, Mercuri LG. Management of temporomandibular joint ankylosis. Oral Maxillofac Surg Clin North Am 2015;27(1):27–35.
52. Anyanechi CE. Temporomandibular joint ankylosis caused by condylar fractures: a retrospective analysis of cases at an urban teaching hospital in Nigeria. Int J Oral Maxillofac Surg 2015;44(8):1027–33.
53. Xiang GL, Long X, Deng MH, et al. A retrospective study of temporomandibular joint ankylosis secondary to surgical treatment of mandibular condylar fractures. Br J Oral Maxillofac Surg 2014;52(3):270–4.
54. Yan YB, Duan DH, Zhang Y, et al. The development of traumatic temporomandibular joint bony ankylosis: a course similar to the hypertrophic nonunion? Med Hypotheses 2012;78(2):273–6.
55. Yan YB, Liang SX, Shen J, et al. Current concepts in the pathogenesis of traumatic temporomandibular joint ankylosis. Head Face Med 2014;10:35.
56. Arakeri G, Kusanale A, Zaki GA, et al. Pathogenesis of post-traumatic ankylosis of the temporomandibular joint: a critical review. Br J Oral Maxillofac Surg 2012; 50(1):8–12.
57. Sidebottom AJ. Post-traumatic management of condylar fracture complications. J Oral Biol Craniofac Res 2022;12(2):284–92.
58. Bera RN, Anand Kumar J, Kanojia S, et al. How far we have come with the Management of Condylar Fractures? A Meta-Analysis of Closed Versus Open Versus Endoscopic Management. J Maxillofac Oral Surg 2022;21(3):888–903.
59. Yao S, Zhou J, Li Z. Contrast analysis of open reduction and internal fixation and non-surgical treatment of condylar fracture: a meta-analysis. J Craniofac Surg 2014;25(6):2077–80.
60. Hackenberg B, Lee C, Caterson EJ. Management of subcondylar mandible fractures in the adult patient. J Craniofac Surg 2014;25(1):166–71.
61. Sporniak-Tutak K, Janiszewska-Olszowska J, Kowalczyk R. Management of temporomandibular ankylosis–compromise or individualization–a literature review. Med Sci Monit 2011;17(5):RA111–6.
62. Schneider M, Erasmus F, Gerlach KL, et al. Open reduction and internal fixation versus closed treatment and mandibulomaxillary fixation of fractures of the mandibular condylar process: a randomized, prospective, multicenter study with special evaluation of fracture level. J Oral Maxillofac Surg 2008;66(12): 2537–44.
63. He D, Cai Y, Yang C. Analysis of temporomandibular joint ankylosis caused by condylar fracture in adults. J Oral Maxillofac Surg 2014;72(4):763.e1–7639.
64. Boffano P, Benech R, Gallesio C, et al. Current opinions on surgical treatment of fractures of the condylar head. Craniomaxillofac Trauma Reconstr 2014;7(2): 92–100.
65. Vesnaver A. Open reduction and internal fixation of intra-articular fractures of the mandibular condyle: our first experiences. J Oral Maxillofac Surg 2008;66(10): 2123–9.
66. Park MW, Eo MY, Seo BY, et al. Gap arthroplasty with active mouth opening exercises using an interocclusal splint in temporomandibular joint ankylosis patients. Maxillofac Plast Reconstr Surg 2019;41(1):18.
67. Zhi K, Ren W, Zhou H, et al. Management of temporomandibular joint ankylosis: 11 years' clinical experience. Oral Surg Oral Med Oral Pathol Oral Radiol Endod 2009;108(5):687–92.

68. Bae SS, Aronovich S. Trauma to the Pediatric Temporomandibular Joint. Oral Maxillofac Surg Clin North Am 2018;30(1):47–60.

69. Demianczuk AN, Verchere C, Phillips JH. The effect on facial growth of pediatric mandibular fractures. J Craniofac Surg 1999;10(4):323–8.

70. Zhang L, Wang Y, Shao X, et al. Open reduction and internal fixation obtains favorable clinical and radiographic outcomes for pediatric mandibular condylar fractures. J Stomatol Oral Maxillofac Surg 2021;122(1):18–23.

71. Akkoc MF, Bulbuloglu S. The Treatment Perspective of Pediatric Condyle Fractures and Long-Term Outcomes. Cureus 2022;14(10):e30111.

72. Rahul M, Ashima G, Akshat G. Arrested root growth and concomitant failure of eruption of a developing tooth following open reduction and internal fixation of a pediatric mandibular fracture. J Indian Soc Pedod Prev Dent 2018;36(2):220–2.

73. Sobrero F, Roccia F, Galetta G, et al. Pediatric mandibular fractures: Surgical management and outcomes in the deciduous, mixed and permanent dentitions [published online ahead of print, 2023 Jan 6]. Dent Traumatol 2023. https://doi.org/10.1111/edt.12814.

74. Singh M, Singh RK, Passi D, et al. Management of pediatric mandibular fractures using bioresorbable plating system - Efficacy, stability, and clinical outcomes: Our experiences and literature review. J Oral Biol Craniofac Res 2016;6(2):101–6.

75. Chocron Y, Azzi AJ, Davison P. Management of Pediatric Mandibular Fractures Using Resorbable Plates. J Craniofac Surg 2019;30(7):2111–4.

76. Pontell ME, Niklinska EB, Braun SA, et al. Resorbable Versus Titanium Rigid Fixation for Pediatric Mandibular Fractures: A Systematic Review, Institutional Experience and Comparative Analysis. Craniomaxillofac Trauma Reconstr 2022;15(3):189–200.

Management of Complications and Secondary Deformity After Fractures of the Midface, Orbit, and Upper Third of the Maxillofacial Skeleton

Nima Vahidi, MD[a], Peter Kwak, MD[a], Dimitrios Sismanis, MD[b],
Theodore Schuman, MD[a], Daniel Hawkins, DMD[c],
Thomas S. Lee, MD[a],*

KEYWORDS

- Craniofacial trauma • Complications • Le Fort fractures • Orbital fractures
- Frontal sinus fractures • Naso-orbito-ethmoid fractures

KEY POINTS

- Craniomaxillofacial trauma management is challenging and can become a chronic problem with many downstream complications.
- Complications of facial trauma can manifest immediately or in a delayed fashion and as such these patients often necessitate long-term follow-up.
- Management of acute or delayed complications is best done by an experienced multidisciplinary team with the use of necessary adjuncts, such as neuronavigation, intraoperative imaging, custom implant use, and virtual surgical planning.

INTRODUCTION

Craniomaxillofacial trauma comprises a large portion of injuries seen in emergency rooms and trauma centers. The most common causes historically have been assaults

---

[a] Department of Otolaryngology – Head and Neck Surgery, Virginia Commonwealth University, 1200 East Broad Street, West Hospital, 12th Floor, South Wing, Suite 313, Clinic Box 980146, Academic Box 980237, Richmond, VA 23298-0146, USA; [b] Oculoplastic Surgery, Virginia Oculofacial Surgeons, 1630 WIlkes Ridges Parkway Suite 102, Richmond, VA 23233, USA; [c] Department of Oral and Maxillofacial Surgery, Virginia Commonwealth University, School of Dentistry, Dental Building 1, 521 North 11th Street, Richmond, VA 23298-0566, USA
* Corresponding author. 1200 East Broad Street, West Hospital, 12th Floor, South Wing, Suite 313, Clinic Box 980146, Academic Box 980237, Richmond, VA 23298-0146.
E-mail address: Thomas.lee@vcuhealth.org

Otolaryngol Clin N Am 56 (2023) 1151–1167
https://doi.org/10.1016/j.otc.2023.05.011
0030-6665/23/© 2023 Elsevier Inc. All rights reserved.

(36%), motor vehicle collisions (32%), falls (18%), sports (11%), occupational (3%), and gunshot wounds (2%). Maxillofacial trauma predominantly affects the younger population (ages 20–40 years), with a predilection for males.[1]

Facial injuries are broadly classified into categories including soft tissue, bony skeleton, and dentoalveolar trauma. Bony trauma is typically subdivided based on location into facial thirds including upper third (frontal sinus, orbital roof, anterior skull base), middle third (orbit, nose, maxilla, and zygoma), and lower third (mandible). Bony facial trauma can also be described based on subsites, such as nasal bone, mandible, dentoalveolar, maxilla/Le Fort, zygomaticomaxillary complex (ZMC), naso-orbital-ethmoid (NOE), and frontal sinus.[2]

A strong fundamental understanding of facial anatomy, surgical approaches, and troubleshooting strategies is needed for proper treatment of this patient population. With the complexity of injury patterns and the multifocal nature of trauma, these patients are plagued by complications and the need for revision surgeries. Here we highlight common fracture patterns of the midface and upper face, along with early and late/postoperative complications and possible management strategies.

LE FORT FRACTURES
Early Complications

A common complication across all Le Fort fractures is malocclusion. Most notorious for resulting in malocclusion are type I Le Fort fractures, which manifest with early contact at the molars resulting in an anterior open bite secondary to the pull of the lateral and medial pterygoid muscles. Type II fractures can result in step-offs, facial asymmetries, and infraorbital nerve paresthesias. Type III Le Fort injury complications include palpable step-offs, facial asymmetries, oral and nasal bleeding, cerebrospinal fluid (CSF) leak, trigeminal nerve damage, and a host of ocular-related injuries.[3,4]

Complications are managed with early (<2 weeks) operative intervention. Maxillomandibular fixation is a useful adjunct to aid in the repair of occlusal deficits. We also advocate for three-dimensional (3D) imaging reconstructed from computed tomography (CT) scans to aid in the preoperative planning process.

Late and Postoperative Complications

Common delayed or postoperative complications result from improperly repaired fractures and can lead to malocclusion and facial asymmetry. Improper reduction can also lead to malunion or nonunion of the bony fragments. Other notable complications include sinusitis (particularly maxillary sinusitis), septal deviation if the fracture involves maxillary crest, cosmetic deformity, hardware failure, or wound breakdown (Table 1). The best way to avoid delayed complications is achieving a healthy wound bed with a good anatomic reduction at the time of the initial surgery. Small bony fragments or devitalized tissues should be debrided from the wound and larger fragments should be rigidly fixated at multiple points. This patient population can manifest with related complications many years following the initial injury.

Long-term complications are typically related to hardware failure and infection.[5,6] For preoperative planning, updated imaging (CT maxillofacial without contrast, 1-mm cuts, with 3D reconstruction) and use of a multidisciplinary team approach are beneficial for this patient population.

Hardware failure is typically related to improper plate use, poor adaptation, inadequate reduction, or poor intraoral gingival mucosal incision closure. If the site of hardware exposure has achieved bony union, 6 to 8 weeks after surgery in the setting of normal bone healing, hardware is removed safely unless the area is missing structurally

Table 1
Early, late, and postoperative complications of Le Fort fractures

Le Fort Fractures	
Early	**Late/Postoperative**
Bleeding	Malunion
Malocclusion	Nonunion
Cranial nerve injury	Hardware failure
CSF rhinorrhea	Facial asymmetry
Orbital hematoma	Infection
Diplopia	Sinusitis
Extraocular muscle entrapment	Nasolacrimal injury
Telecanthus	Osteomyelitis

crucial bone. If malunion or nonunion is present, bone should be debrided until healthy vascularized bone is encountered. In rare instances, bone grafting may be warranted if there is notable loss along the vertical midface buttresses. If there is a significant malalignment resulting in malocclusion and malunion, osteotomies may be necessary to reduce the fracture with the application of new hardware.

Representative Case

Fig. 1 shows a patient presenting with a type I Le Fort fracture with malocclusion and anterior open bite showing preoperative and postoperative position following a revision Le Fort I osteotomy to restore class 1 occlusion. In this case, bone grafting was necessary to provide continuity at the piriform buttresses. Preoperative and postoperative 3D imaging demonstrates the restoration of premorbid class 1 occlusion.

ZYGOMATICOMAXILLARY FRACTURES
Early Complications

Patients with ZMC fractures often present with pain, epistaxis, diplopia, subconjunctival hemorrhage, and periorbital edema and ecchymosis. Another common manifestation of injury is loss of lateral cheek projection from posterior or medial displacement of the malar eminence. Initial evaluation of this injury pattern may prove difficult because soft tissue edema can mask this deformity.

Displaced zygomatic fractures can also cause trismus secondary to compression of the zygomatic arch on the coronoid process or temporalis muscle. Many of the early manifestations of injury resolve with time; however, significant injuries with functional problems, such as trismus or diplopia, may require surgical intervention.[7]

Late and Postoperative Complications

Delayed or postoperative complications following ZMC fractures include malunion or nonunion, maxillary sinusitis, facial asymmetry from malar flattening, and poor cosmesis. Improper reduction over time can lead to malar flattening or increased facial width.[8] Given the close proximity to the orbit, visual disturbances can manifest in the posttreatment phase including enophthalmos, ectropion, canthal malpositioning, and long-standing diplopia (**Table 2**).[9]

Common complications of ZMC fractures that necessitate revision surgery include cosmetic deformity (malar flattening) and persistent diplopia secondary to inadequate orbital volume. Malar flattening is caused by inadequate bony reduction and posterior-

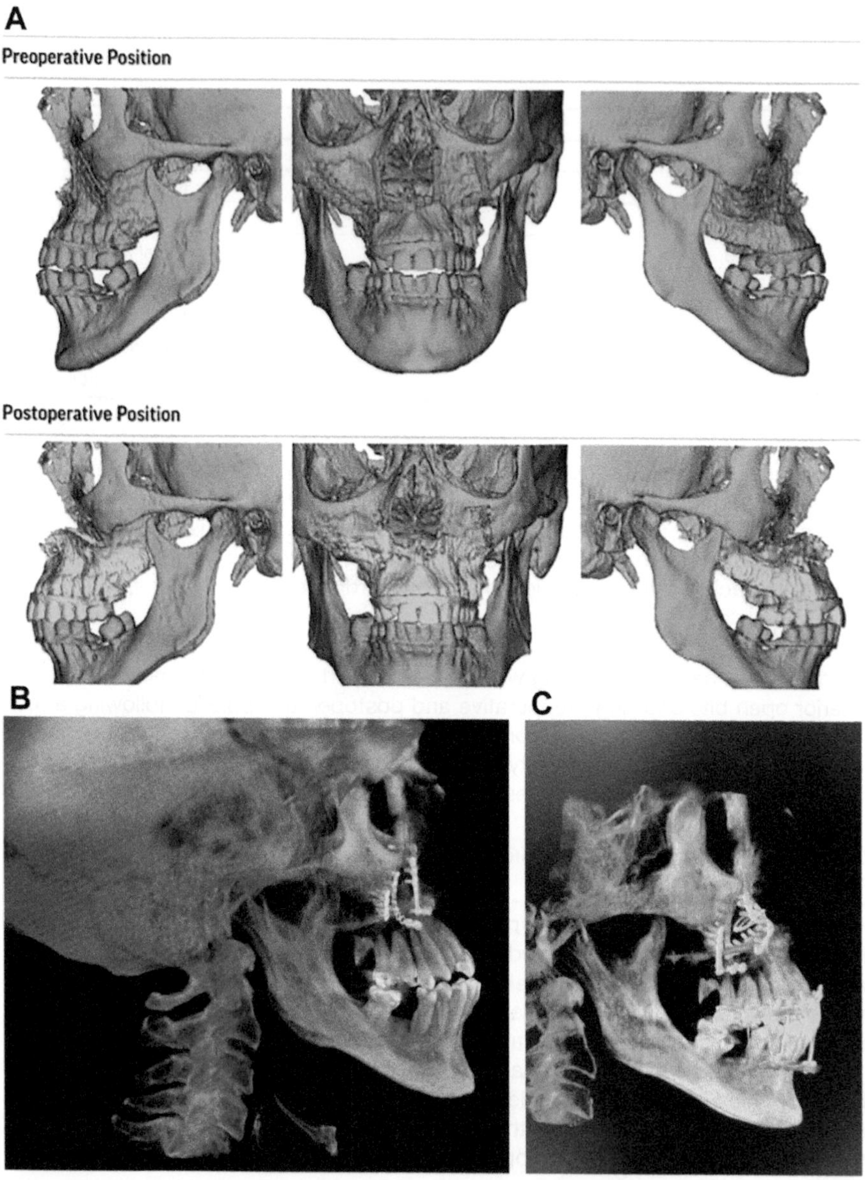

A

Preoperative Position

Postoperative Position

B   **C**

Fig. 1. Patient with a type I Le Fort fracture presenting with malocclusion and an anterior open bite. (*A*) Preoperative and postoperative position following a revision Le Fort I osteotomy to restore class 1 occlusion. (*B*) Preoperative and (*C*) postoperative 3D imaging demonstrating the restoration of premorbid class 1 occlusion.

medial displacement of the malar segment. It is critical to achieve a near anatomic reduction at the time of initial intervention to avoid this long-term complication. It is important during surgery to use the zygomatic buttresses to reestablish premorbid coaptation including the curvature of the zygomaticomaxillary suture line, the lateral orbital rim borders, and the infraorbital rim. Although not always visualized the

Table 2	
Early, late, and postoperative complications of ZMC fractures	
Zygomaticomaxillary Fractures	
Early	**Late/Postoperative**
Swelling	Malunion
Facial asymmetry	Nonunion
Visual disturbances	Hardware failure
Trismus	Facial asymmetry
Diplopia	Sinusitis
	Diplopia
	Enophthalmos
	Hypoglobus

zygomaticosphenoid suture provides the single most accurate assessment of bony reduction. In addition to visual confirmation, palpation and comparison with the contralateral malar eminence may prove useful.

The decision for surgical intervention to correct cosmetic deformity in ZMC fractures largely depends on the presence or absence of additional functional deficits, such as trismus or diplopia. In instances of isolated malar flattening without functional deficits one can improve the cosmetic outcome by increasing the bony or soft tissue volume of the malar eminence. Options for restoring malar projection include the use of nonvascularized bone grafts, fat grafting, temporary or permanent fillers, or customized implants. Customized implants have become more widely accepted in recent years, although the implantable material and approach is still debated.[10]

In instances of poor visualization, surgical neuronavigation or intraoperative CT scanning can also be useful especially when natural bony landmarks have been disturbed. These adjuncts are particularly useful in bilateral injury patterns because direct comparison with the undisturbed side is not possible. However, these adjuncts may not be available in all instances and should not be relied on as such.

Hardware infection in all facial trauma poses a challenging problem but particularly in ZMC fractures because of the 3D nature of the malar segment. In these instances, it is important to remove the existing hardware and prioritize anatomic reduction and restoration of function. We also recommend against implantation of new hardware or custom implants in an actively infected wound bed. Long-standing reduction defects may necessitate the use of osteotomies, which increases the surgical complexity but is necessary to achieve an optimal result. When performing osteotomies to improve bony reduction we recommend addressing the zygomaticomaxillary (ZM), zygomaticofrontal (ZF), and infraorbital rim segments before the orbital floor, lateral orbital wall, and medial orbital wall. This proves additionally important in instances of implant use because the prosthesis cannot otherwise be properly secured.

Representative Case

Fig. 2 shows a 37-year-old woman who presented to our institution with a remote history of ZMC fracture now with persistent diplopia, localized infection with a draining fistula, and chronic maxillary sinusitis. On preoperative imaging, inferiorly displaced orbital floor implant, uncorrected lateral orbital wall defect because of poor ZMC bone reduction along the ZS suture line, orbital implant migration medially obstructing the maxillary sinus drainage, and right-sided malar flattening are demonstrated. The patient underwent a revision open reduction internal fixation of a right-sided ZMC fracture with use of neuronavigation. The defect was approached through a combination

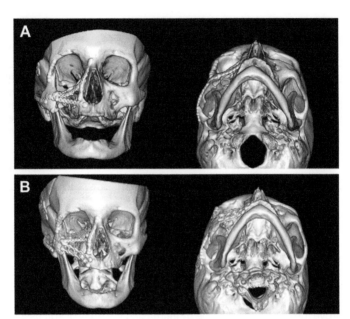

Fig. 2. Patient with a remote history of ZMC fracture develops persistent diplopia, a drain-ing fistula, and chronic maxillary sinusitis. (*A*) On preoperative imaging, inferiorly displaced orbital floor implant, uncorrected lateral orbital wall defect caused by poor ZMC bone reduction along the ZS suture line, orbital implant migration medially obstructing the maxil-lary sinus drainage, and right-sided malar flattening are demonstrated. (*B*) The patient un-derwent a revision open reduction internal fixation of a right-sided ZMC fracture with use of neuronavigation.

of methods including preexisting lateral eyelid laceration, lateral brow incision, trans-conjunctival incision with lateral canthotomy, and an intraoral maxillary vestibular inci-sion. We performed an osteotomy at the anterior zygomatic arch, lateral orbital rim, zygomaticosphenoid suture, and zygomaticomaxillary sutures to mobilize the segment. Reduction was performed beginning with the lateral orbital rim along the zygomaticosphenoid suture followed by the zygomaticomaxillary suture. Positioning was confirmed with intraoperative navigation. After the malar segment was appropri-ately fixated, we proceeded with orbital floor and medial orbital wall defect reconstruc-tion. An endoscopic maxillary mega-antrostomy was also performed. Postoperatively the patient had resolution of diplopia, no further signs of infection, and improved malar projection and cosmesis.

ORBITAL FRACTURES

The primary objective with orbital repair is restoration of orbital volume and premorbid orbital architecture. Several surgical approaches exist for obtaining surgical exposure including the subciliary, infraorbital, transconjunctival, and transcaruncular approaches. It is the senior authors' (D.S., T.S.L.) preference to use the transconjunctival incision with or without a concurrent lateral canthotomy for most repairs. Orbital floor defect repair often necessitates the use of autologous or alloplastic material to reconstruct.

Traditional indications for primary surgical repair include hypoglobus, enophthal-mos of greater than 2 mm, oculocardiac reflex, optic nerve compression, diplopia from entrapment, or cosmetic deformity. Quantitative metrics also exist for surgical repair including greater than 50% of the orbital floor or fractures greater than 3 cm² of the floor or greater than 2 cm² along the medial orbit.[11,12] Persistent oculocardiac reflex and orbital apex syndrome often necessitate emergent surgical intervention.[13] For those cases without immediate surgical needs, surgical correction is recommended between 1 and 2 weeks of injury once the orbital edema has gone down, or electively in the future. Orbital exploration during the first week may prove challenging because of the soft tissue edema of the orbital contents and may lead to a suboptimal reduction.

Early Complications

Complications following orbital floor fractures can unfortunately be common and include edema, ecchymosis, diplopia, extraocular movement limitations, hypoglobus, enophthalmos, hypoesthesia, oculocardiac reflex, and blindness. Vision loss is among the most serious complications following orbital trauma and has been reported in roughly 7.1% to 7.8% of patients.[14] Vision loss following orbital fracture repair is fortunately much rarer, with one major study citing a rate of 0.3%.[15] Many of these manifestations of partial or total vision compromise warrant urgent evaluation and possible surgical intervention depending on the underlying cause.

Late and Postoperative Complications

Long-term complications following orbital trauma include diplopia, enophthalmos, hypoglobus, ectropion, hardware failure, chronic maxillary sinusitis, sinonasal cutaneous fistula, hypoesthesia or paresthesia, retraction, entropion or ectropion, and lagophthalmos (**Table 3**). Persistent enophthalmos has been documented in 27% of postoperative patients, and diplopia in between 8% and 52%. Restoring orbital volume and restoring premorbid reduction are important in avoiding the postoperative complications of enophthalmos and hypoglobus. Poorly repaired orbital fractures often present with a constellation of findings including eyelid retraction with ectropion or entropion, motility disruption, and hyperglobus.

Hardware failure can accompany structural shortcomings manifesting with hardware malpositioning, migration, extrusion, or infection. Focusing on proper plate coaptation and fixation to healthy structural bone is important in avoiding the potentially devastating complications of hardware failure.

Important pitfalls to avoid include appropriately sizing the length and width of the implant as to contact the ledges of the fracture. Placing a short implant can lead to

Table 3	
Early, late, and postoperative complications of orbital fractures	
Orbital Fractures	
Early	**Late/Postoperative**
Diplopia	Diplopia
Subconjunctival hemorrhage	Hypoglobus
Retinal edema	Enophthalmos
Enophthalmos	Ectropion
Hypoglobus	Infraorbital nerve dysfunction
Hyphema	Entropion
Vision loss	Sinonasal fistula
Retrobulbar hematoma	Chronic sinusitis
Globe rupture	
Orbital apex syndrome	

the implant angulating into the maxillary sinus and placing an implant that is too long can either become visible in the lower eyelid or impinge the posterior orbital structures. The orbital floor implant should always sit behind the infraorbital rim as to avoid hardware visibility or discomfort. Placement of the implant behind the rim also allows for better contour and adaptation to the natural "s"-shaped curvature of the orbital floor. Selecting the appropriate width implant is equally as important as selecting the correct length. The medial most aspect of the implant should be in contact with remaining medial orbital wall that is stable or medial buttress of maxilla. If there is inadequate medial orbital wall support, the implant can migrate into the nasal cavity causing obstruction of the maxillary ostiomeatal complex.

Another common cause of downstream complications is inadequate reduction of the orbital floor fracture and orbital contents leading to asymmetric orbital floor positioning. This is avoided by dissecting in a subperiosteal plane along the orbital floor and the medial orbital wall until stable bone is encountered. In rare instances a transcaruncular approach may be necessary to gain entry to the medial orbital wall when stable bone is not encountered.

We advocate for the use of Medpor or Medpor-titanium hybrid implants and recommend avoiding titanium-only implants when possible. Titanium-only implants can lead to abnormal scarring of the periorbital soft tissues, which leads to significant soft tissue ingrowth, scar contracture, and limitation in extraocular movements. The Medpor implants typically form a surrounding capsule that avoids the undesired complications of the titanium-only implants. The soft tissue ingrowth also makes it exceedingly difficult to remove titanium-only implants in the future should the need arise. It is also important with these implants that they are secured with at least one screw anteriorly along the infraorbital rim to prevent migration.

The placement of orbital incisions is extremely important to obtain exposure when necessary but also limit complications. Ectropion and retraction can occur in the setting of subciliary or transconjunctival incisions, whereas entropion is unique to transconjunctival incisions. Transconjunctival approaches cause cicatricial entropion by traumatizing the tarsus and conjunctiva. This is directly related to the initial incision and as such it is our preference to tent the palpebral conjunctiva by grasping it in the inferior fornix and incising several millimeters below the inferior tarsal borders. Alternatively, some surgeons evert the lid margin with a retractor and use a Jaeger plate against the internal aspect of the orbital rim to retropulse the orbital contents and then incise the conjunctiva and retractors directly at the orbital rim. There is no harm in cutting the retractors at this level. We have found with this approach that if the implant is fixated to the anterior aspect of the orbital rim, this incision acts as another tethering point for the eyelid and globe and releasing cicatrix and salvaging conjunctiva is particularly difficult. It is important that medially the incision is directed toward the caruncle and away from the nasolacrimal apparatus.

Representative Case

A 60-year-old man presented with right-sided facial pain, swelling, with concerns for orbital hardware infection (**Fig. 3**). He had a history of right-sided orbital floor and ZMC fractures and repair 1-year prior at another institution. On evaluation, he was noted to have right maxillary tenderness and on nasal endoscopy had exposed hardware in the middle meatus and diplopia. Coronal imaging demonstrated a right-sided orbital floor implant. The medial aspect of the implant migrated inferiorly and was noted to be obstructing the maxillary os and exposed to the nasal cavity contents. The orbital implant was removed in a revision surgery. Decision was made to not alter the existing ZMC fracture that shows signs of minor malar flattening and facial widening because

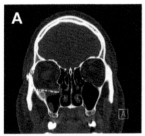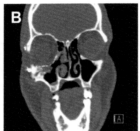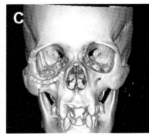

Fig. 3. Patient presented with right-sided facial pain and swelling, and concern for orbital hardware infection. (*A*) Coronal imaging demonstrates a right-sided orbital floor implant. The medial aspect of the implant has migrated inferiorly and was noted to be obstructing the maxillary os and exposed to the nasal cavity contents. The orbital implant was removed in a revision surgery. Decision was made to not alter the existing ZMC fracture that shows signs of minor malar flattening and facial widening because cosmesis was not a major concern to the patient. The orbital volume correction was completed with a new, properly shaped and positioned orbital floor implant. Postoperative imaging (*B*) coronal and (*C*) 3D reconstruction.

cosmesis was not a major concern to the patient. The orbital volume correction was completed with a new, properly shaped and positioned orbital floor implant.

NASO-ORBITO-ETHMOID FRACTURES

NOE fractures are commonly classified by the Markowitz and Manson classification system, which is a three-tier classification system based on severity of injury to the medial canthal tendon. Type I fractures manifest with a single large fractured segment and an intact medial canthal tendon. Type II fractures demonstrate comminution but maintain an intact medial canthal tendon. Type III fractures demonstrate comminution and avulsion of the medial canthal tendon.[16]

The goal of operative intervention for NOE fractures is multifactorial. The primary goal is reduction of the nasal root to restore premorbid soft tissue contour of the glabella. Secondarily, it is important to restore the intercanthal distances and attaching the medial canthus to a stable landmark. Finally, reestablishing the medial vertical buttress system is important to ensure facial symmetry and stability.

Type I fractures can often be treated with closed nasal reduction, fixation of the NOE bone segment, and external splinting. Type II and III fractures often necessitate bony fixation and medial canthal repositioning. For moderately displaced fractures we recommend fixation of the inferior segment of the NOE segment via a maxillary vestibular approach. If there is persistent instability involving the superior NOE segment a modified lynch incision or preexisting laceration approach may be necessary to obtain adequate access for proper fixation. We recommend a bicoronal approach for concurrent NOE and anterior table frontal sinus fractures.

Many surgical options exist for restoration of the medial canthal distance and repositioning the medial canthal tendons. We recommend the use of titanium miniplates anchored to the NOE bone segments and suture suspension (4–0 clear Nylon) to secure the medial canthus to the plates with several redundant sutures placed. It is our opinion that the use of transnasal wiring is technically complex and results in undesirable crusting within the nasal cavity and increases the risk for downstream hardware infections.

Early Complications

Patients with NOE fractures may present with cosmetic deformity, telecanthus, diplopia, epistaxis, and nasal obstruction. These patients typically warrant early operative repair (<2 weeks) to reestablish projection and symmetry of the NOE region.[4] Higher velocity injuries can result in a different spectrum of injuries including cribriform plate fractures and nasolacrimal duct injuries leading to CSF leaks or epiphora. High-impact injuries typically call for a multidisciplinary approach involving colleagues in ophthalmology and neurosurgery.

Late and Postoperative Complications

Long-term and postoperative complications of NOE fractures include telecanthus, enophthalmos, saddle nose deformity, nasal obstruction, epiphora, and hardware failure (**Table 4**). Revision procedures often pose a significant challenge and as such it is important when possible to address any deficits or dysfunction in the early posttraumatic period. The NOE region is one of the most challenging from a reconstructive standpoint and it may require multistage surgeries.

  NOE fractures can result in a multitude of complications and as such it is important to organize and prioritize the treatment plan. For isolated NOE fractures restoring the medial vertical buttress is of utmost importance because it restores midface structural stability. Following reestablishment of the architecture of the NOE region it is then important to reestablish medial canthus attachments and restore lacrimal duct patency if obstructed. Restoring nasal airway patency is another important functional consideration and any cosmetic concerns that need to be addressed. In NOE fractures with concurrent skull base injury, the skull base injury is prioritized, and the NOE fracture may need to be addressed in a staged fashion. If CSF leak is present it should be treated appropriately, either managed conservatively or with operative intervention. Posterior table fractures that are comminuted may necessitate cranialization. Anterior table fractures should be addressed with the same priority as restoring the medial vertical buttress system because it is an important architectural landmark.

Representative Case

A 59-year-old man presented to our emergency room following a firework explosion to the face (**Fig. 4**) with resulting bilateral type 3 NOE fractures, bilateral Le Fort I fractures, and lacerations along nose and upper lip. The patient underwent bilateral NOE repairs through the existing nasal laceration and bilateral Le Fort I

Table 4	
Early, late, and postoperative complications of NOE fractures	
Naso-orbito-ethmoid Fractures	
Early	**Late/Postoperative**
Anosmia	Cosmetic nasal deformity
Epiphora	Telecanthus
Visual disturbances	Enophthalmos
CSF leak	Anosmia
Telecanthus	Epiphora
Midface retrusion	Dacryocystitis
Telecanthus	Forehead paresthesia
	Pseudohypertelorism
	Hardware failure

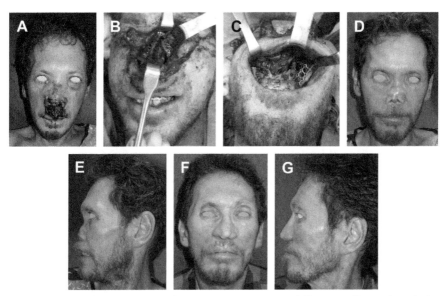

Fig. 4. A 59-year-old man presented to our emergency room following a firework explosion to the face (*A*) with resulting bilateral type 3 NOE fractures, bilateral Le Fort I fractures, and lacerations along nose and upper lip. (*B*) Patient underwent bilateral NOE repairs through the existing nasal laceration and (*C*) bilateral Le Fort I fracture repair through a standard maxillary vestibular incision. The goal of the initial surgery was to reduce and fixate the midfacial bones, restore medial canthus positioning bilaterally, and provide skin coverage for the underlying bone and hardware. (*D, E*) Postoperative the patient had achieved appropriate symmetry and projection of the midface and placement of the medial canthal tendons. He did, however, develop a significant saddle nose deformity because of loss of native nasal cartilage. (*F, G*) In a staged fashion we performed a paramedian forehead flap with a dorsal onlay rib graft to rebuild the dorsal L-strut while de-epithelializing the native nasal skin to provide a foundation on which to build. The patient also underwent bilateral melolabial flaps in a staged fashion to recreate nasal ala symmetry and projection. At this time the patient is satisfied with his results and no longer interested in further interventions.

fracture repair through a standard maxillary vestibular incision. A Prolene suture secured the left medial canthus to the miniplate, resuspending the detached canthal tendon. The right medial canthal tendon was secured in a similar fashion. Given the large mucosal defect we elected to reconstruct the nose in a staged fashion and avoid the risk of cartilage graft failure. The goal of the initial surgery was to reduce and fixate the midfacial bones, restore medial canthus positioning bilaterally, and provide skin coverage for the underlying bone and hardware. Postoperatively the patient achieved appropriate symmetry and projection of the midface and placement of the medial canthal tendons. He did, however, develop a significant saddle nose deformity because of loss of native nasal cartilage. In a staged fashion we performed a paramedian forehead flap with a dorsal onlay rib graft to rebuild the dorsal L-strut while de-epithelializing the native nasal skin to provide a foundation on which to build. The patient also underwent bilateral melolabial flaps in a staged fashion to recreate nasal ala symmetry and projection. At this time the patient is satisfied with his results and no longer interested in further interventions.

FRONTAL SINUS FRACTURES

The frontal sinuses offer protection to the anterior cranial fossa in traumatic situations.[17] The force required to fracture the frontal sinuses is greater than any other facial bone.[18] Frontal sinus traumas are classified based on the involvement of the anterior table, posterior table, and frontal recess. In recent years, there has been a shift in management of frontal sinus fractures with a greater tendency for frontal sinus preservation because of advancement of minimally invasive, endoscopic sinus surgery.[19]

Early Complications

Early complications of frontal sinus trauma occur within the first 6 months of injury. These include facial deformity, headaches, CSF leak, infection, meningitis, pneumocephalus, and supraorbital or supratrochlear nerve injury.

Wound infections and soft tissue deficits are managed conservatively with culture-directed antibiotics and local wound care.[20] Facial nerve and sensory deficits should be monitored closely; most resolve over time.[21] Contour irregularities are addressed with in-office filler to camouflage if there is minimal risk of sinus mucosal exposure or operative repair to restore frontal projection. Hydroxyapatite injection to the frontal sinus region should be avoided because it is associated with a high rate of infection if there is sinus mucosal exposure.[22]

Late and Postoperative Complications

Long-term and postoperative complications of frontal sinus trauma include chronic sinusitis, mucocele, contour irregularities, osteomyelitis, and frontal sinus cutaneous fistula. Many frontal sinus complications can manifest months to years following the initial injury.[23] Many of these complications stem from frontal sinus mucosal trauma and nasofrontal duct injury. Patients with downstream symptoms of headache, facial pain, nasal discharge, or obstruction should be further evaluated for potential complications (**Table 5**).

Mucocele and mucopyoceles can form many years following a frontal sinus injury often secondary to obstruction of the nasofrontal outflow tract or incomplete removal of frontal sinus mucosa. As such, it is imperative at the time of the initial surgery to remove the mucosal lining of the frontal sinus, in particular the mucosa along the lateral margins of the frontal sinus and along the frontal sinus roof. Improved visualization of the sinus by removing bony ledges of the anterior table allows for a more thorough debridement. Given that these lesions can manifest years later, surveillance CT imaging is recommended. Postobstructive disease is a common late complication and may manifest as chronic sinusitis or mucocele formation. Conservative measures

Table 5	
Early, late, and postoperative complications of frontal sinus fractures	
Frontal Sinus Fractures	
Early	**Late/Postoperative**
Infection	Sinusitis
Contour irregularity	Mucocele
Frontal headaches	Mucopyocele
Cerebrospinal fluid leak	Contour irregularity
Meningitis	Osteomyelitis
Supraorbital/supratrochlear nerve injury	Frontal sinus cutaneous fistula
	Hardware failure
	Frontal headaches

often fail to resolve these symptoms. Endoscopic frontal sinusotomy is an important and highly efficacious strategy for the management of this patient population.[19]

Hardware failure is another common long-term complication that often necessitates intervention. Hardware failure can manifest in different ways, including skin or soft tissue breakdown, osteomyelitis, or concurrent sinusitis. It is important at the time of initial surgery to achieve an appropriate bony reduction and to provide adequate soft tissue coverage for underlying hardware. This is especially important when using existing lacerations to obtain access to the defect because there may be poor soft tissue coverage overlying the implanted hardware and may result in delayed hardware exposure. The pericranial flap with its blood supply based on the noninjured side is a versatile flap that is used for soft tissue coverage, frontal sinus obliteration, or anterior skull base reconstruction.

Representative Case

A 48-year-old man presented to our clinic with a history of intermittent forehead swelling (**Fig. 5**). He had a remote history of a frontal sinus fracture repair with frontal sinus obliteration performed at another institution. Preoperative axial and sagittal imaging demonstrated opacification of the frontal sinuses, mucocele, and hardware failure. Surgical indications included frontal sinus mucocele, subperiosteal abscess, and hardware failure. At time of surgery the patient was noted to have significant forehead and facial swelling indicative of underlying abscess and hardware infection. A titanium mesh was used to restore the anterior table defect. Care was taken to secure the plate

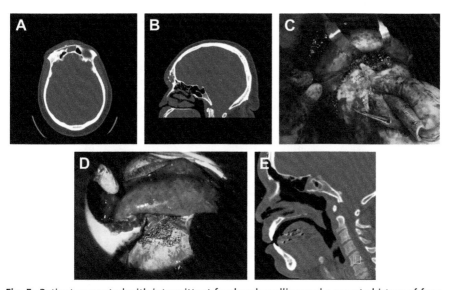

Fig. 5. Patient presented with intermittent forehead swelling and a remote history of frontal sinus fracture repair and frontal sinus obliteration. Preoperative imaging (*A*) axial and (*B*) sagittal demonstrated opacification of the frontal sinuses, mucocele, and hardware failure. Surgical indications included frontal sinus mucocele, subperiosteal abscess, and hardware failure. At time of surgery the patient was noted to have significant forehead and facial swelling indicative of underlying abscess and hardware infection. (*C*) A titanium mesh was used to restore the anterior table defect (*D*). Care was taken to secure the plate to healthy bone. (*E*) Postoperative CT scan sagittal, showing restoration of the anterior table and aeration of frontal sinus.

to healthy bone. The overlying skin flap was noted to be thin and irregular because of long-standing soft tissue infection and as such we elected to place a nonvascularized strip of temporalis muscle to cover the hardware and restore appropriate forehead contour on external evaluation. Postoperative sagittal CT scan showing restoration of the anterior table and aeration of frontal sinus.

A 62-year-old man presented with nasal congestion and left-sided periorbital edema (**Fig. 6**). He had a remote history of facial trauma 20 years previously and had undergone facial plating of the left frontal sinus. On evaluation he was noted to have left forehead tenderness and edema. Sagittal and coronal imaging demonstrated a bony fragment obstructing the left frontal sinus outflow tract and sinus opacification. Hardware was removed and devitalized soft tissues and infection were debrided.

PANFACIAL FRACTURES

Panfacial injuries involving the upper face, midface, and cranial vault pose a particular challenge for reconstructive surgeons. These cases initially are overwhelming, particularly when assessing the multitude of injuries and considering the treatment

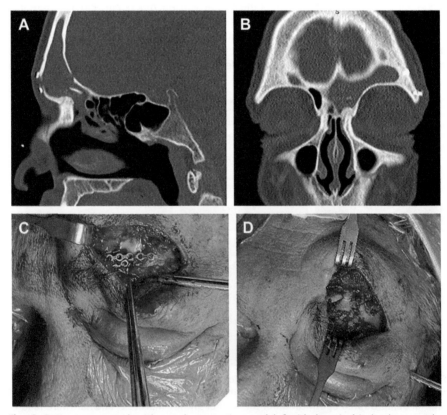

Fig. 6. Patient presented with nasal congestion and left-sided periorbital edema and a distant history of frontal sinus fractures and hardware placement. Imaging (*A*) sagittal and (*B*) coronal demonstrates a bony fragment obstructing the left frontal sinus outflow tract and sinus opacification. (*C*) Intraoperative photograph demonstrating purulence surrounding the frontal sinus hardware. (*D*) Following the removal of hardware and debridement of devitalized soft tissues and infection.

plan. Here we highlight our experience with a particularly challenging patient that presented as a trauma alert to our institution with a shotgun blast to the middle and upper face. This case demonstrates the importance of prioritizing issues and treating patients in a systematic and staged fashion. Panfacial injuries and gunshots are notorious for high complication rates and as such we discuss our recommendations.

A 17-year-old man presented to our institution as a trauma alert following a shotgun blast to the mid and upper face. On primary evaluation the patient was noted to have a large soft tissue and bony defect of the midface and anterior cranial vault. The priority in this case was securing the airway and assessing neurologic status. Neurosurgery intervened emergently and performed a decompressive craniotomy. The patient was noted at this time to have exposed frontal brain parenchyma; bilateral injuries to the anterior cranial vault; defects of the frontal bone and NOE region; and a full-thickness soft tissue defect of the scalp, forehead, and nose (**Fig. 7**A).

Maxillofacial intervention was delayed until the patient had improved from a neurologic standpoint and was communicative. It was only after neurologic improvement

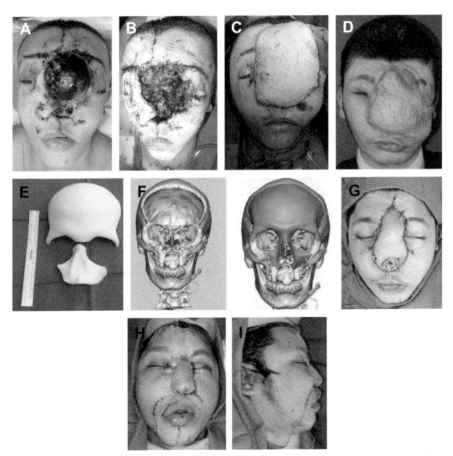

Fig. 7. (*A*) Patient with a shotgun blast injury to the midface and skull base with full-thickness soft tissue and bony defects. (*B-I*) Reconstructive stages illustrating complex skull base and midface reconstruction with custom implants and microvascular free flaps.

and a discussion with the patient and family that we decided to pursue aggressive and definitive reconstructive surgery. Our initial surgical goal was providing skin and soft tissue coverage over the exposed frontal brain parenchyma and addressing the CSF leak (**Fig. 7**B). The facial skeleton was not addressed during our initial surgical intervention. The skull base defect was reconstructed with hinged soft tissue to provide support and prevent herniation of the frontal lobe contents into the nasal cavity. The soft tissue reconstruction at this stage was performed with an anterolateral thigh (ALT) free flap (**Fig. 7**C).

The next surgical intervention was focused on restoring bony architectural support for the anterior cranial vault, frontal bone, and midface (**Fig. 7**D). Given the extent of bone loss the decision was made that free flap reconstruction was not a viable option. We proceeded with the creation of a custom Medpor implant for the cranial vault and midface, which was placed through a bicoronal fashion sandwiched within the ALT soft tissues (**Fig. 7**E, F). The next stage of surgery involved debulking the ALT soft tissues and restoring the intercanthal distance by performing bilateral medial canthoplasty. The medial canthal tendons were secured to the buried Medpor implant with nonabsorbable suture (**Fig. 7**G).

The fourth stage focused on midface reconstruction with the use of an osteocutaneous radial forearm free flap and autologous rib grafting (**Fig. 7**H, I). Given the nature of his soft tissue injury the paramedian forehead flap was not a viable option. The radial forearm flap was used to provide an external skin lining and a nasal mucosal lining. Despite multiple attempts at restoring nasal patency, we were unable to successfully maintain nasal airflow. Ultimately, we performed revision surgery to achieve an acceptable cosmetic result for the external nose while still maintaining soft tissue coverage of the underlying hardware.

CLINICS CARE POINTS

- For complex orbital, skull base or panfacial fracture cases, neuronavigation can be a useful tool to help identify fractures and may assist in bone reduction.

- Virtual surgical planning with customized implants can be useful for reduction and fixation of complex fractures with poor bony references and can also decrease operative time.

- Long-term follow-ups may be of benefit to check for delayed complications, such as mucocele formation or delayed hardware failure.

DISCLOSURE

None.

REFERENCES

1. Singaram M, SV G, Udhayakumar RK. Prevalence, pattern, etiology, and management of maxillofacial trauma in a developing country: a retrospective study. J Korean Assoc Oral Maxillofac Surg 2016;42(4):174–81.
2. Allareddy V, Allareddy V, Nalliah RP. Epidemiology of facial fracture injuries. J Oral Maxillofac Surg 2011;69(10):2613–8.
3. Lozada K, Kadakia S, Abraham MT, et al. Complications of midface fractures. Facial Plast Surg 2017;33(6):557–61.
4. Morris LM, Kellman RM. Complications in facial trauma. Facial Plast Surg Clin North Am 2013;21(4):605–17.

5. Hernandez Rosa J, Villanueva NL, Sanati-Mehrizy P, et al. Review of maxillofacial hardware complications and indications for salvage. Craniomaxillofac Trauma Reconstr 2016;9(2):134–40.
6. Salentijn EG, van den Bergh B, Forouzanfar T. A ten-year analysis of midfacial fractures. J Cranio-Maxillo-Fac Surg 2013;41(7):630–6.
7. Barry C, Coyle M, Idrees Z, et al. Ocular findings in patients with orbitozygomatic complex fractures: a retrospective study. J Oral Maxillofac Surg 2008;66(5): 888–92.
8. Olate S, Lima SM Jr, Sawazaki R, et al. Surgical approaches and fixation patterns in zygomatic complex fractures. J Craniofac Surg 2010;21(4):1213–7.
9. Ellis E 3rd, Reddy L. Status of the internal orbit after reduction of zygomaticomaxillary complex fractures. J Oral Maxillofac Surg 2004;62(3):275–83.
10. Jones CM, Schmalbach CE. Zygomaticomaxillary fractures. Facial Plast Surg Clin North Am 2022;30(1):47–61.
11. Kunz C, Sigron GR, Jaquiery C. Functional outcome after non-surgical management of orbital fractures: the bias of decision-making according to size of defect: critical review of 48 patients. Br J Oral Maxillofac Surg 2013;51(6):486–92.
12. Sung YS, Chung CM, Hong IP. The correlation between the degree of enophthalmos and the extent of fracture in medial orbital wall fracture left untreated for over six months: a retrospective analysis of 81 cases at a single institution. Arch Plast Surg 2013;40(4):335–40.
13. Kim BB, Qaqish C, Frangos J, et al. Oculocardiac reflex induced by an orbital floor fracture: report of a case and review of the literature. J Oral Maxillofac Surg 2012;70(11):2614–9.
14. Mellema PA, Dewan MA, Lee MS, et al. Incidence of ocular injury in visually asymptomatic orbital fractures. Ophthalmic Plast Reconstr Surg 2009;25(4): 306–8.
15. Girotto JA, Gamble WB, Robertson B, et al. Blindness after reduction of facial fractures. Plast Reconstr Surg 1998;102(6):1821–34.
16. Markowitz BL, Manson PN, Sargent L, et al. Management of the medial canthal tendon in nasoethmoid orbital fractures: the importance of the central fragment in classification and treatment. Plast Reconstr Surg 1991;87(5):843–53.
17. Lee TS, Kellman R, Darling A. Crumple zone effect of nasal cavity and paranasal sinuses on posterior cranial fossa. Laryngoscope 2014;124(10):2241–6.
18. De Boer HH, Van der Merwe AE, Soerdjbalie-Maikoe VV. Human cranial vault thickness in a contemporary sample of 1097 autopsy cases: relation to body weight, stature, age, sex and ancestry. Int J Legal Med 2016;130(5):1371–7.
19. Arnold MA, Tatum SA 3rd. Frontal sinus fractures: evolving clinical considerations and surgical approaches. Craniomaxillofac Trauma Reconstr 2019;12(2):85–94.
20. Cleveland PW, Smith JE. Complications of facial trauma of the fronto-orbital region. Facial Plast Surg 2017;33(6):581–90.
21. Metzinger SE, Metzinger RC. Complications of frontal sinus fractures. Craniomaxillofac Trauma Reconstr. 2009;2(1):27–34.
22. Verret DJ, Ducic Y, Oxford L, et al. Hydroxyapatite cement in craniofacial reconstruction. Otolaryngol Head Neck Surg 2005;133(6):897–9.
23. Rohrich RJ, Hollier LH. Management of frontal sinus fractures. Changing concepts. Clin Plast Surg 1992;19(1):219–32.

Pediatric Head and Neck Trauma

Sara Bressler, MD, Lisa Morris, MD*

KEYWORDS

• Pediatric facial trauma • Pediatric neck trauma • Mandible fracture • Orbital fracture

KEY POINTS

- Traumatic injury to the head and neck is more common in children than adults, however, only 5-15% of all facial fractures occur in children.
- When fractures occur in the pediatric patient, there is a risk of growth restriction and subsequent facial deformity, not only from the initial injury but also from iatrogenic injury during treatment.
- Outcomes depend on the age of patient, site of injury, management options, and subsequent growth.

INTRODUCTION

Traumatic injury to the head and neck is more common in children than adults, however, only 5-15% of all facial fractures occur in children.[1] This decreased fracture risk is due to the increased stability and inherent flexibility of the pediatric craniofacial skeleton. When fractures occur in the pediatric patient, there is a risk of growth restriction and subsequent facial deformity, not only from the initial injury but also from iatrogenic injury during treatment. The purpose of this article is to guide the head and neck trauma surgeon in decision making for the treatment of pediatric head and neck trauma with an emphasis on facial fracture management.

CRANIOFACIAL TRAUMA
Anatomic Differences between Children and Adults

Children are not just small adults. This population has unique anatomic characteristics that bring challenges and increased risk to management. The pediatric facial skeleton is constantly changing from birth to adulthood, allowing for varying fracture patterns and fracture management strategies. A child's face is composed of more cartilage,

Louisiana State University Health Sciences Center-New Orleans, 533 Bolivar Street Suite 566, New Orleans, LA 70112, USA
* Corresponding author.
E-mail address: Lmor17@lsuhsc.edu

Otolaryngol Clin N Am 56 (2023) 1169–1182
https://doi.org/10.1016/j.otc.2023.05.012

a higher ratio of periosteum, compliant sutures, and bone that is less mineralized than adults. This allows the bone to bend rather than break. The pediatric facial skeleton is also more stable due to the lack of pneumatization of the paranasal sinuses and unerupted teeth in the mandible and maxilla.

The skull-to-face ratio is approximately 8:1 at birth which decreases to 2.5:1 in adulthood.[2] The larger skull-to-face ratio in young children results in frontal protrusion of the cranium with relative retrusion of the face, placing the forehead at increased risk for frontal impact injury.[1,3] As such, the cranium is at higher risk of injury and younger children are more likely to sustain frontal bone fractures compared to midface or mandibular fractures. Vertical development of the face occurs with paranasal sinus formation, dental maturation, dental eruption, and mandibular growth at the condylar growth centers.[4] This increases the risk of midface and mandible fractures as the child matures.

The paranasal sinuses are diminutive at birth. The maxillary sinuses develop first, extending inferiorly to the level of the nasal floor by about age 12 and reaching adult size by 16 years of age.[5,6] The ethmoid sinuses begin development at birth and reach their full size by age 12.[7] As growth continues, the medial orbital wall, or lamina papyracea, becomes progressively thinner until it is "paper thin" in adulthood and thus more susceptible to fracture.[8] The frontal sinus begins to develop around 1-2 years of age and becomes identifiable radiographically around 4-7 years old when the sinuses are pneumatized to the level of the orbital roof. Pneumatization continues into adolescence with a rapid post-pubertal growth phase between 13 and 16 years, with pneumatization not complete until adulthood.[5]

Primary (deciduous) dental eruption begins around 6 months of age with the full eruption of the 20 deciduous teeth by 2.5 years of age. The primary dentition is relatively stable until root resorption beings to occur so that the deciduous crowns begin to loosen and exfoliate around age 6. The mixed dentition stage occurs between 6 and 12 years of age. Full eruption of the permanent dentition occurs by ages 12-14 years with third molars (wisdom teeth) erupting in early adulthood.[4,9] The presence of developing tooth buds increases the maxillary and mandibular stability and decreases the risk of displaced fractures. Both tooth buds and unerupted teeth are at risk of injury with plate and screw placement and bone-anchored interdental fixation devices.

Evaluation

All pediatric trauma patients should be evaluated based on the Advanced Trauma Life Support (ATLS) protocol with both primary and secondary surveys.[10] Pediatric patients are at an increased risk for rapid decompensation compared to adults (**Table 1**) and should be stabilized prior to beginning the secondary survey in which

Table 1
Anatomic and physiologic characteristics that lead to a higher risk of decompensation in pediatric patients[10,18]

Hypovolemia	Lower blood volume, higher cardiac output, children tolerate a loss of up to 1/3 of total blood volume before developing hypotension due to the ability to compensate and maintain systolic blood pressure
Hypothermia	Larger body surface area-to-overall mass ratio
Hypoxia	Increased metabolic rate and oxygen demand. May be difficult to intubate with smaller airway, short neck, anteriorly positioned larynx, and a more "floppy airway"

craniofacial injuries are evaluated. A systematic examination is important to avoid omitting possible injury sites, especially in the pediatric population as obtaining a complete history and physical examination can be challenging depending on their developmental stage. The patient may be unable to verbalize symptoms, cooperate with examination or work up, and may not comply with recommended treatment. Sedation or general anesthesia may be required for complete evaluation. A careful intraoral examination is necessary to evaluate for mucosal and dental injuries. Accounting of all teeth is critical, as they may represent an airway foreign body. It is critical to evaluate for concomitant injuries associated with pediatric trauma, especially intracranial and cervical spine injuries as they can result in severe neurologic sequela and mortality.[3,11–13] Neurosurgery, ophthalmology, and dental consultation should be obtained when indicated. Medical providers should also be vigilant for non-accidental trauma (NAT) in this vulnerable population. Fifty percent of NAT cases will result in head or neck injuries.[1,9] Young children are at the greatest risk with nearly a third of victims found to be less than 2 years of age.[14]

Imaging

Computed tomography (CT) scanning is the gold standard for evaluating facial fractures.[15] Both maxillofacial CT and Cone beam CT (CBCT) are the ideal modalities for the most comprehensive evaluation of the facial skeleton.[16] CT imaging with multiplanar reformatting and three-dimensional (3D) volume rendering of image data (**Fig. 1**) provides precise anatomic details, allowing for accurate diagnosis and detailed treatment planning.[1,4,11,17] Periapical and occlusal radiographs provide high-resolution images for the evaluation of dental injury. Panoramic tomography (Panorex) can evaluate both dental and bone injury of the mandible. This is especially useful for the evaluation of dentoalveolar fractures and dental injury.[10] Chest and abdominal x-rays are needed if teeth, dental fragments, or dental appliances are not accounted for to ensure they were not aspirated or swallowed.[9] Digital photography can assist with patient and caregiver education, preoperative versus postoperative monitoring, and future reconstructive planning if needed.[18,19]

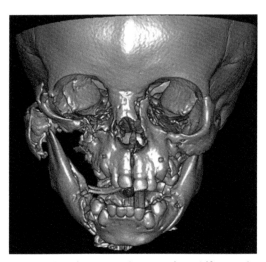

Fig. 1. 3D CT scan reconstruction demonstrating complex midface and mandibular fractures in a 6 month old unrestrained passenger involved in a motor vehicle crash.

MANAGEMENT OF CRANIOFACIAL TRAUMA
Soft Tissue

Soft tissue injuries occur in association with facial fractures 29-56% of the time.[17] These injuries can be easily overlooked as they may be covered in dried blood, bandages, c-collar, or other obstructing items. Soft tissue injuries in the pediatric population are treated similarly to adults. All wounds should be cleaned, and thorough exploration of any laceration is needed to evaluate for damage to the underlying structures.[19] Dissolvable sutures are optimal for pediatric soft tissue repair as they do not require compliance with removal.[10] Surgeons should consider that when permanent suture material or staples are used, young children may require sedation or general anesthesia to remove.

Facial Fractures

Pediatric facial fractures are unique and often distinct from those seen in adults. Pediatric facial fracture patterns vary by age, depending on the stage of facial maturation and mechanism of injury (**Box 1**).[3] Green stick fractures, which are incomplete fractures of the bone, are typical in the pediatric population. These fractures are often minimally displaced and require less intervention.[20] Pediatric patients have a rapid healing potential and therefore any surgical intervention should be considered earlier than adults, often within 7 days after injury.[4,7]

There is no definitive protocol for the treatment of pediatric facial fractures, but there is consensus for more conservative treatment whenever possible to avoid growth disturbances.[21] Treatment options depend on fracture location, severity of dislocation, facial anatomy, stage of dental eruption, and developmental stage of the patient. Morisada and colleagues[22] posit that the aim of pediatric facial fracture treatment is to match the degree of fracture stabilization needed to the patient's age and healing potential while preventing inadvertent iatrogenic consequences to unerupted teeth and

---

Box 1
Age-based epidemiological factors with pediatric facial trauma[9,17]

Preschool age (Birth-5 years)
- Lowest incidence of facial fractures.
- Falls are the leading cause of trauma as they are learning to walk and become mobile.
- Below age 2, injuries to the frontal region and orbital roof are more common.
- These are typically low-impact, low-velocity forces, leading most commonly to isolated, nondisplaced fractures.

School age (6–12 years)
- Mixed dentition stage and have increasing pneumatization of the paranasal sinuses.
- Second highest risk of facial fractures, typically due to MVCs, play, and bike riding.
- With increased activity and less parental supervision, school-aged children have a higher risk of midface and mandible fractures with condylar fractures being the most common.
- Orbital floor fractures become more common than the orbital roof with the expansion of the maxillary sinus.

Teenage (13–18 years)
- Highest incidence of facial fractures as they gain more independence, start driving, engage in contact sports, and interpersonal violence is more common.
- Rapid facial growth occurs in a forward and downward direction, leading to the lower 1/3 of the face at highest risk for injury.
- With the permanent dentition fully erupted, the mandible is at increased risk with fracture patterns becoming more adult-like.
- Management of facial fractures is more similar to adults.

growth centers. In as much, a minimalist approach is often recommended in preschool and school aged children. If significant displacement is present, fracture reduction is necessary to bring bone fragments close enough in order for remodeling to occur. As patients approach skeletal maturity, open reduction with internal fixation (ORIF) is performed more frequently.[23] Children 13 years of age and older have more adult-like anatomy with the full eruption of their dentition, and management typically follows adult facial trauma protocols.[4]

Growth Disturbance

For all ages, the goals of fracture management are to restore form and function. In the pediatric population, it is equally important to prevent future growth disturbance, which can lead to significant facial deformity and dysfunction. Growth disturbance can occur from the initial injury or from iatrogenic causes during the fracture management. Disruption of growth centers, limitation of suture growth, scar formation by stripping of periosteum, decreased vascularity, and misalignment of fracture segments can lead to subsequent facial deformity. The head and neck trauma surgeon should consider the severity of the fracture and the amount of displacement, along with the age and stage of dental development of the patient. Facial growth after trauma can be unpredictable and long-term follow-up is necessary to monitor functional and aesthetic outcomes.[18] Patients and families should be educated regarding the risk of growth disturbances and the sequela of long-term facial deformity.

Upper facial trauma
Cranial bone, frontal bone, and orbital roof fractures. Frontal bone and frontal sinus fractures account for 5% of all pediatric facial fractures and are more common in preschool aged patients.[24] Without a pneumatized frontal sinus, these fractures can easily extend along the orbital roof as well. Given the large amount of force required to fracture the frontal bone, patients need to be evaluated for concomitant traumatic brain injury.[25] The incidence of intracranial complications, including pneumocephalus and intracranial hemorrhage, is reported to range from 35% to 64%.[18] Physicians should therefore have a low threshold to screen for signs and symptoms of neurologic impairment and to obtain dedicated imaging of the brain to rule out underlying injury.

Only about 10% of frontal bone and frontal sinus fractures require surgical intervention.[26,27] Surgical intervention may be required if there are displaced bone fragments causing symptoms or structural damage, compromise to the orbital contents, or the involvement of brain tissue.[27] Regardless of the patient's age or fracture pattern, a multidisciplinary approach with neurosurgery and ophthalmology should be pursued given the close anatomic relationship of these structures. In young children without a pneumatized frontal sinus, frontal bone fractures are considered skull fractures. Skull fractures are generally treated non-operatively but should be managed according to neurosurgical guidelines with considerations for patients with focal neurologic symptoms, increasing intracranial pressures or cerebral compression, persistent cerebrospinal fluid leak, dural laceration, or pneumocephalus.[28] As the frontal sinus begins to pneumatize, the treatment goals become similar to adults with a focus on the patency of the nasofrontal outflow tract. In the absence of nasofrontal outflow tract obstruction or CSF leak, patients with posterior table fractures can be observed.[29] Fractures extending into the orbital roof are often managed conservatively via a multidisciplinary approach. Immediate surgical intervention should be pursued if there is clinical evidence of entrapment, enophthalmos, or vertical orbital dystopia. If surgical intervention is warranted for depressed or displaced fracture segments, open reduction and internal fixation (ORIF) is performed through existing lacerations, superolateral orbital rim approach, or a coronal approach.[27] For children in whom bony remodeling and frontal sinus development is still occurring, observation can be a reasonable option, even for significantly depressed or displaced fractures, with no resulting long term cosmetic deformity or identifiable radiographic evidence of injury.[30] A rare but serious intracranial complication is the growing skull fracture, which is most common in children under 2 years of age.[11] As the brain pulsates, this fracture line enlarges, leading to the resorption of the adjacent bone and herniation of brain parenchyma through the fracture. This requires dural repair and ORIF of the cranial bone.[31]

Midface trauma

Orbital fractures. The need for surgical intervention in pediatric orbital fractures depends largely on the patient's clinical findings at the time of presentation, underscoring the importance of the physical examination. Entrapment of the extraocular muscles is one of the most common complications associated with orbital floor fractures and is an indication for emergent operative intervention. Entrapment occurs when there is a greenstick fracture of the orbital floor that is initially displaced however due to the elastic nature of pediatric bones, the fracture segment snaps back to its initial position, trapping orbital contents within the fracture.[7,17,32] This trap door or "white eye" fracture is more common in pediatric patients than in adults, especially those under 6 years of age.[33] Clinical findings include diplopia, ophthalmoplegia, pain on upward gaze, and activation of the oculocardiac reflex (a vagally mediated reflex that results in bradycardia, nausea/vomiting, and syncope, with the potential for asystole).[34] Nausea and vomiting are predictive of tissue entrapment with a positive predictive value of 80-83%.[34,35] The fracture site and soft tissue findings of fat and/or muscle herniation may be difficult to identify on a CT scan. When radiographic findings do not correlate with clinical findings, orbital entrapment should remain a clinical diagnosis.[18,36,37] Entrapment is considered a surgical emergency and timely treatment is critical to prevent muscle ischemia and permanent impairment in extraocular movement.[33]

Large orbital floor defects can be managed conservatively with good outcomes in this population. If the periosteum and the ligamentous support of the globe remain intact, a sufficient sling may be present to support the orbital contents.[7,8] Losee and colleagues[38] found that among patients with large bony defects (greater than 50% in length or width or with severe displacement) treated conservatively, 70% did not develop enophthalmos, and the remaining developed mild enophthalmos that was only noted only by the surgeon and not the family. Patients treated conservatively should be reevaluated after 1-2 weeks, once edema has resolved, to assess for diplopia and enophthalmos. In general, diplopia that is present on exam will either remain the same or improve but will rarely, if ever, worsen.[39] Persistent central gaze diplopia may warrant surgical intervention. Surgical approaches to the orbit are similar to those used in adults. Historically, autologous grafts such as cartilage or bone were used for reconstruction due to their biocompatibility, however these have fallen out of favor because of prolonged operative times and significant donor site morbidity.[40] Over time, surgeons have made the switch to allografts due to their availability, durability, and increased tensile strength.[32]

Nasal and naso-orbito-ethmoid fractures. Nasal fractures are common and often go undiagnosed. In the pediatric nose, the cartilaginous septum extends from the nasal tip to the skull base. As the child matures, portions of the septum progressively ossify. Small deviations of the flexible cartilage can lead to larger deformities as the nose grows. The nasal bones are separated by a midline suture, making them easy to displace with trauma.[41] Treatment is determined based on the presence of deformity, therefore imaging for an isolated nasal injury is not needed. Closed nasal reduction with external fixation is preferred.[7] Ideal timing for fracture reduction is in the first 5-7 days once the swelling has improved.[17] Intranasal evaluation is imperative in all facial fractures to evaluate for septal hematomas, which should be drained immediately and splinted to prevent the reaccumulation of blood.[7,18] Naso-orbito-ethmoid (NOE) fractures are evaluated for traumatic telecanthus (increased intercanthal width of the eyes), shortened width of the palpebral fissures and a saddle nose deformity. While rare in children, they can lead to devastating deformity that is difficult to repair secondarily. NOE fractures typically follow adult management protocols, if they are severe and deformity is present.[7]

ZMC/zygoma/LeFort fractures. Complex midface fractures are rare in children due to poorly pneumatized maxillary sinuses, unerupted dentition, and an undeveloped maxillary buttress system. Conservative treatment is typically all that is needed; however, displaced or unstable fractures will require maxillomandibular fixation (MMF) and/or open reduction internal fixation (ORIF).[18]

Lower facial trauma

Dental injuries. Twenty-five percent of school-aged children experience dental trauma.[10] Goals of treatment during *primary dentition* is to (1) avoid injury to the developing permanent tooth and (2) avoid severe malocclusion from displaced dentoalveolar segment. Injury to *permanent dentition* requires prompt referral to a dentist or endodontist and may require splinting.[9] If avulsion of a primary tooth occurs, it should not be replaced.[17] Avulsion of a permanent tooth requires replantation as soon as possible to avoid the desiccation of the periodontal ligament. Avoid placing the tooth in water or allowing it to dry. It can be stored in saline, the buccal vestibule or milk prior to replantation. The time out of the dental socket is critical with death of periodontal ligament cells beginning within 30 minutes. Once replantation is performed, a flexible splint will hold it in position for 2-4 weeks and close dental follow up is needed. Root canal therapy is typically initiated within 2 weeks after replantation. Replantation occurring after 60 minutes has a poor prognosis but should still be considered for esthetics and alveolar bone contour. The tooth can be extracted at a later date with time for planning dental replacement options.[10]

Dentoalveolar fractures. Dentoalveolar fractures occur when the alveolar process and teeth fracture as a unit. Treatment requires reduction into appropriate position and stabilization with the splinting of the teeth, arch bar, dental wiring, or miniplate fixation of the alveolar bone (**Fig. 2**). Endodontic treatment should be performed within 2 weeks of injury to help maintain the viability of the tooth.[10]

Mandible fractures. Mandible fractures account for a third of all facial fractures in the pediatric population.[22] Management of pediatric mandibular fractures is more conservative than adults with fewer MMF and ORIF procedures. The goals of treating mandibular fractures are to re-establish normal jaw function and occlusion, maintenance of facial symmetry, and to minimize growth restriction.[42] Mandible fractures in young children are less common and are more likely to be a greenstick fracture with minimal displacement.[22] The majority of mandibular fractures in younger pediatric patients are treated conservatively with a soft/no chew diet, close observation, and avoidance of physical activities (17, 4, 42). Minor malocclusion is tolerated as it will correct with future growth and remodeling.[7,22] Operative treatment is minimized due to the increased risks of injuring the developing dentition and causing growth disruption. However, complex fractures and significantly displaced fractures need to be reduced and immobilized. If

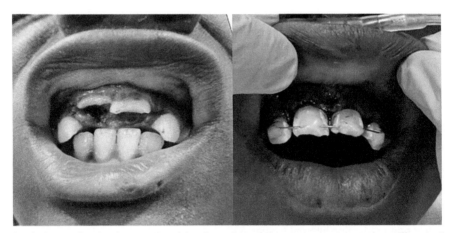

Fig. 2. Dentoalveolar fracture involving intrusion of the permanent central maxillary incisors and displacement the overlying alveolar bone. The dentition and alveolar bone were repositioned and stabilized with a light wire passive splint.

in primary or early mixed dentition, tooth buds or unerupted dentition are at risk for injury with ORIF. Immobilization can be achieved with specialized MMF techniques (see later in discussion). Once in the mixed dentition stage, monocortical plating may be placed along the inferior border of the mandible with care to avoid unerupted permanent dentition and the inferiorly positioned inferior alveolar nerve. With the full eruption of the permanent dentition, the treatment protocol begins to mirror adult mandible fracture algorithms.[3] Pediatric bone healing is more rapid and therefore surgical intervention should be expedited within the first week and the duration of rigid MMF should be minimized (1–3 weeks). Fractures typically heal within 3-4 weeks.[43] General guidelines of mandibular fracture are listed in **Box 2**.

Fixation
Maxillomandibular fixation. MMF is utilized as a closed reduction method as it holds the upper and lower jaws in stable occlusion while fractures of the midface and/or lower face heal. MMF offers a shorter operative period with decreased soft tissue

---

Box 2
General guidelines for the management of pediatric mandibular fractures

- Pediatric mandible fractures without significant displacement or malocclusion are managed conservatively with a soft/no chew diet.

- Condylar fractures and subcondylar fractures without significant malocclusion can be managed with a soft diet and early range of motion.[42] Ankylosis of the temporomandibular joint is more common in children, resulting in impaired jaw function.[17] For severe injury, a brief period (7–10 days) of MMF may be appropriate.[4]

- Displaced fractures at other sites of the mandible can be managed with a 2.0 mm miniplate over the lower mandibular border with monocortical screw fixation (mixed dentition) or acrylic lingual splinting (primary dentition).[4]

- MMF is less traumatic to the periosteum and may have less risk for growth restriction.

- Teenagers in the permanent dentition stage can be treated with standard adult mandibular fracture protocols with both MMF or ORIF as indicated.

trauma.[44] The ideal method of MMF is dependent upon the child's dental stage. During the primary or mixed dentition stages MMF can be challenging. Techniques avoiding damage to developing tooth buds should be utilized, such as circummaxillo-mandibular wiring, acrylic splints, or MMF with dental wires (ie, Risdon wires or ivy loops).[18] In mixed dentition standard Erich arch bars and wiring techniques may be difficult due to loose or missing teeth. Once permanent teeth have erupted, intermax-illary fixation (IMF) screws, Hybrid arch bars, and standard Erich arch bars may be employed. Extended periods of MMF increase the risk of temporomandibular joint (TMJ) ankylosis in children. Typically, a duration of 1-2 weeks of rigid MMF followed by guiding elastics is recommended.[42] Complications associated with MMF include weight loss, poor oral hygiene, psychosocial difficulties, and communication difficulties.[42]

Plating. Displaced fractures that will not self-correct with compensatory growth require ORIF with accurate and stable reduction to prevent functional or aesthetic impairment.[11] Both titanium and resorbable plating systems are options for fixation. Titanium plating systems have been the standard of care with well-accepted dura-bility, versatility, and biocompatibility.[45,46] Disadvantages to titanium include hard-ware migration though growing bone, palpability, imaging interference, temperature sensitivity, stress shielding, chronic pain, and infection.[45] To minimize these complica-tions, many surgeons advocate for return to the operating room for removal of titanium hardware once fractures are healed. Biodegradable plating systems are composed of polymers of polylactic acid (PLA) and polyglycolic acid (PGA) and resorb by hydrolysis. These plates maintain their strength for 4-10 weeks during fracture healing and degra-dation occurs over 1-4 years.[42,47] Disadvantages to resorbable plates are that a heat source is required for the bending of the plates and pretapping is needed for screw placement. Resorbable hardware is not as strong as titanium hardware, but they have been demonstrated to be equally effective in upper and midface fracture repair and pediatric mandible fractures without increased complications.[45–47]

There is no consensus regarding the need for titanium hardware removal, the period of time it should remain, or the ages at which it should be removed. Arguments for the removal of titanium plates are to minimize the risk of growth restriction and plate migra-tion. Plate migration occurs by natural jaw growth with the deposition of bone on the buccal cortex and resorption on the lingual cortex. The plate is progressively covered with new bone. To avoid this, plate removal is recommended between 1 and 3 months.[4,22] A systematic review of upper and midfacial fractures by Pontell and col-leagues[46] found that titanium hardware had a higher complication rate compared to resorbable hardware (27% versus 17%) and 87% of the titanium group underwent a second surgery for elective hardware removal, with none in the resorbable group.

NECK TRAUMA

Penetrating and blunt neck trauma is rare in the pediatric population but may be more devastating due to smaller anatomy and proximity of critical structures. There is a high risk for injury to the aerodigestive tract, vasculature, nerves, vertebrae, and cervical spine. Vascular and airway injuries can be life-threatening. Stone and colleagues[48] reviewed the National Trauma Data Bank from 2008 to 2012 for pediatric penetrating neck trauma and found a mortality rate of 5.6%, with "vascular injury" and "hypoten-sion upon presentation to the mergency department" variables independently associ-ated with death. Laryngotracheal trauma is the second most common cause of mortality in head and neck trauma after intracranial injury.[49]

Table 2	
Hard and soft signs indicating the need for emergent operative treatment in pediatric penetrating neck trauma	
Hard Signs	**Soft Signs**
Shock	Dyspnea
Active hemorrhage	Hemoptysis
Pulsatile bleeding or expanding hematoma	Nonexpanding hematoma
Audible bruit or palpable thrill	Laceration greater than 2 cm
Airway compromise	Hoarseness
Stridor	Dysphagia
Wound bubbling	Odynophagia
Massive subcutaneous emphysema	Palpable crepitus
Difficulty swallowing secretions	Voice change
Neurological deficits	

Initial management of pediatric neck trauma is similar to adults. Early diagnosis and treatment are paramount with initial evaluation during the primary assessment of the ATLS protocol. The airway is stabilized with endotracheal intubation or emergent tracheostomy, if indicated. "Hard" and "soft" signs found on examination that require immediate neck exploration are listed in **Table 2**.[48,50,51] In patients found to be stable, CT imaging is performed followed by flexible fiberoptic laryngoscopy if there is any concern for laryngeal injury.[49,52] For the evaluation of penetrating neck trauma, the neck is divided into 3 anatomical zones: zone I–from the clavicle to the cricoid cartilage, zone II–from the cricoid cartilage to the angle of the mandible, and zone III–from the angle of the mandible to the base of the skull. Penetrating injuries to zone II are most common.[51] There has been a recent shift of guidelines in the adult protocol in the management of zone II penetrating injury that has been adopted in the pediatric population as well. Mandatory surgical exploration has changed to selective neck exploration based on physical examination and CT angiogram in stable patients.[48,50,51] The work up is dependent upon the CT findings and extent of injury, which may include flexible or rigid tracheobronchoscopy, esophagoscopy, other operative interventions, swallow study, or esophagram.[48,51,52] Management of laryngotracheal and esophageal injuries vary depending on the nature of the injury and the clinical stability of the patient. Treatment options range from observation to intubation to surgical intervention depending on the site of injury, need for positive pressure ventilation, and the presence of concomitant injuries. Esophageal perforations should be ruled out prior to enteral feeding to avoid mediastinitis.[52]

SUMMARY

The head and neck trauma surgeon should be aware of the differences in the management of pediatric patients and that a more conservative approach is favored when possible. Outcomes depend on the age of the patient, site of injury, management options, and subsequent growth. Children must be followed over an extended period of time to monitor both immediate complications with healing but also long-term complications with subsequent facial growth.

CLINICS CARE POINTS

- The pediatric population has a lower rate of facial fractures due to the increased stability and inherent flexibility of the pediatric craniofacial skeleton

- CT imaging with multiplanar reformatting and three-dimensional (3D) volume rendering of image data is ideal for evaluation of facial fractures, offering precise anatomic details for accurate diagnosis and detailed treatment planning
- There is no definitive protocol for treatment of pediatric facial fractures, but there is consensus for more conservative treatment whenever possible to avoid growth disturbances
- Children 13 years of age and older have more adult-like anatomy with full eruption of their dentition, and management typically follows adult facial trauma protocols
- Pediatric patients have a rapid healing potential and therefore any surgical intervention for a facial fracture should be considered earlier than adults, often within 7 days after injury
- Facial growth after trauma can be unpredictable and long term follow up is necessary to monitor functional and aesthetic outcomes
- In young children without a pneumatized frontal sinus, frontal bone fractures are considered skull fractures
- The majority of mandibular fractures in younger pediatric patients are treated conservatively with a soft/ no chew diet, close observation, and avoidance of physical activities
- Penetrating and blunt neck trauma is rare in the pediatric population but may be more devastating due to smaller anatomy and proximity of critical structures
- The work up for pediatric penetrating neck trauma is dependent upon the CT/CTA findings and extent of injury, with selective neck exploration only when indicated

CONFLICTS OF INTERESTS

L. Morris MD has no disclosures or conflicts of interests.
S. Bressler MD has no disclosures or conflicts of interests.

REFERENCES

1. Alcalá-Galiano A, Arribas-García IJ, Martín-Pérez MA, et al. Pediatric facial fractures: children are not just small adults. Radiographics 2008;28(2):441–618.
2. Maisel H. Postnatal growth and anatomy of the face. In: Mathog RH, editor. Maxillofacial trauma. Baltimore, MD: Williams & Wilkins; 1984. p. 21–38.
3. Berlin RS, Dalena MM, Oleck NC, et al. Facial fractures and mixed dentition - what are the implications of dentition status in pediatric facial fracture management? J Craniofac Surg 2021;32(4):1370–5.
4. Wolfswinkel EM, Weathers WM, Wirthlin JO, et al. Management of pediatric mandible fractures. Otolaryngol Clin North Am 2013;46(5):791–806.
5. Lee S, Fernandez J, Mirjalili SA, et al. Pediatric paranasal sinuses-Development, growth, pathology, & functional endoscopic sinus surgery. Clin Anat 2022;35(6): 745–61.
6. Whyte A, Boeddinghaus R. The maxillary sinus: physiology, development and imaging anatomy. Dentomaxillofac Radiol 2019;48(8):20190205 [Epub 2019 Aug 13. Erratum in: Dentomaxillofac Radiol. 2019 Sep 10;:20190205c. PMID: 31386556; PMCID: PMC6951102].
7. Braun TL, Xue AS, Maricevich RS. Differences in the management of pediatric facial trauma. Semin Plast Surg 2017;31(2):118–22.
8. Oppenheimer AJ, Monson LA, Buchman SR. Pediatric orbital fractures. Craniomaxillofac Trauma Reconstr 2013;6(1):9–20.
9. Olynik CR, Gray A, Sinada GG. Dentoalveolar trauma. Otolaryngol Clin North Am 2013;46(5):807–23.

10. Sosovicka M, DeMerle M. AdolescenT OROFACIAL TRAUma. Dent Clin North Am 2021;65(4):787–804.

11. Lim RB, Hopper RA. Pediatric facial fractures. Semin Plast Surg 2021;35(4): 284–91. Published 2021 Oct 11.

12. Shah J, Wang F, Ricci JA. Concomitant cervical spine injuries in pediatric maxillofacial trauma: an 11 year review of the national trauma data bank. J Oral Maxillofac Surg 2023;81(4):413–23.

13. Xun H, Lopez J, Darrach H, et al. Frequency of cervical spine injuries in pediatric craniomaxillofacial trauma. J Oral Maxillofac Surg 2019;77(7):1423–32.

14. U.S. Department of Health & Human Services, Administration for Children and Families, Administration on Children, Youth and Families, Children's Bureau. (2023). Child Maltreatment 2021. Available at: https://www.acf.hhs.gov/cb/data-research/child-maltreatment. Accessed on March 20, 2023.

15. Talwar AA, Heiman AJ, Kotamarti VS, et al. High-resolution maxillofacial computed tomography is superior to head computed tomography in determining the operative management of facial fractures. J Surg Res 2020;256:381–9.

16. Alimohammadi R. Imaging of dentoalveolar and jaw trauma. Radiol Clin North Am 2018;56(1):105–24.

17. Gupta K, Verma N, Katiyar A, et al. A stitch in time saves nine: all about pediatric facial fracture. Natl J Maxillofac Surg 2022;13(1):27–31.

18. Andrew TW, Morbia R, Lorenz HP. Pediatric facial trauma. Clin Plast Surg 2019; 46(2):239–47.

19. Schild S, Puntarelli TR, delaPena M, et al. Facial soft tissue injuries in pediatric patients. Facial Plast Surg 2021;37(4):516–27.

20. Moffitt JK, Wainwright DJ, Bartz-Kurycki M, et al. Factors associated with surgical management for pediatric facial fractures at a level one trauma center. J Craniofac Surg 2019;30(3):854–9.

21. Pereira I, Pellizzer E, Lemos C, et al. Closed versus open reduction of facial fractures in children and adolescents: a systematic review and meta-analysis. J Clin Exp Dent 2021;13(1):e67–74. Published 2021 Jan 1.

22. Morisada MV, Tollefson TT, Said M, et al. Pediatric mandible fractures: mechanism, pattern of injury, fracture characteristics, and management by age. Facial Plast Surg Aesthet Med 2022;24(5):375–81.

23. Segura-Palleres I, Sobrero F, Roccia F, et al. Characteristics and age-related injury patterns of maxillofacial fractures in children and adolescents: a multicentric and prospective study. Dent Traumatol 2022;38(3):213–22.

24. Gassner R, Tuli T, Hächl O, et al. Craniomaxillofacial trauma in children: a review of 3,385 cases with 6,060 injuries in 10 years. J Oral Maxillofac Surg 2004;62(4): 399–407.

25. Pappachan B, Alexander M. Biomechanics of cranio-maxillofacial trauma. J Maxillofac Oral Surg 2012;11(2):224–30.

26. Coon D, Kosztowski M, Mahoney NR, et al. Principles for management of orbital fractures in the pediatric population: a cohort study of 150 patients. Plast Reconstr Surg 2016;137(4):1234–40.

27. Connon FV, Austin SJ, Nastri AL. Orbital roof fractures: a clinically based classification and treatment algorithm. Craniomaxillofac Trauma Reconstr 2015;8(3): 198–204.

28. Lopez J, Pineault K, Pradeep T, et al. Pediatric frontal bone and sinus fractures: cause, characteristics, and a treatment algorithm. Plast Reconstr Surg 2020; 145(4):1012–23.

29. Vu, Anthony T, Patel PA, Chen W, et al. Pediatric frontal sinus fractures: outcomes and treatment algorithm. J Craniofac Surg 2015;26(3):776–81.

30. MacIsaac ZM, Naran S, Losee JE. FACS. pediatric frontal sinus fracture conservative care: complete remodeling with growth and development. J Craniofac Surg 2013;24(5):1838–40.

31. Singhal GD, Atri S, Suggala S, et al. Growing skull fractures; pathogenesis and surgical outcome. Asian J Neurosurg 2021;16(3):539–48.

32. Wei LA, Durairaj VD. Pediatric orbital floor fractures. J AAPOS 2011;15(2):173–80.

33. Bera RN, Tiwari P, Pandey V. Does early treatment of paediatric orbital fracture offer any advantage in terms of post-operative clinical outcomes. J Maxillofac Oral Surg 2022;21(1):25–33.

34. Firriolo JM, Ontiveros NC, Pike CM, et al. Pediatric orbital floor fractures: clinical and radiological predictors of tissue entrapment and the effect of operative timing on ocular outcomes. J Craniofac Surg 2017;28(8):1966–71.

35. Cohen SM, Garrett CG. Pediatric orbital floor fractures: nausea/vomiting as signs of entrapment. Otolaryngol Head Neck Surg 2003;129(1):43–7.

36. Glassman GE, Jackson K, Pontell ME, et al. Pediatric orbital entrapment: radiographic findings and their predictive values. Ann Plast Surg 2021;86(6S):S606–9.

37. Pontell ME, Jackson K, Golinko M, et al. Influence of radiographic soft tissue findings on clinical entrapment in patients with orbital fractures. J Craniofac Surg 2021;32(4):1427–31.

38. Losee JE, Afifi A, Jiang S, et al. Pediatric orbital fractures: classification, management, and early follow-up. Plast Reconstr Surg 2008;122(3):886–97.

39. Chung SY, Langer PD. Pediatric orbital blowout fractures. Curr Opin Ophthalmol 2017;28(5):470–6. PMID: 28797015.

40. Azzi J, Azzi AJ, Cugno S. FRCSC*. Resorbable material for pediatric orbital floor reconstruction. J Craniofac Surg 2018;29(7):1693–6.

41. Morris L. Rhinoplasty in kids: why, how, and when. Curr Otorhinolaryngol Rep 2022;10:155–61.

42. Kao R, Rabbani CC, Patel JM, et al. Management of mandible fracture in 150 children across 7 years in a US tertiary care hospital. JAMA Facial Plast Surg 2019;21(5):414–8.

43. Ellis III, E and Schubert W. 2021. Osteosynthesis in the growing skeleton. AO Surgery Reference, 2nd Ed. Available at: <https://surgeryreference.aofoundation.org/cmf/trauma/mandible/further-reading/osteosynthesis-in-the-growing-skeleton>. Assessed on April 25, 2023.

44. Kao R, Campiti VJ, Rabbani CC, et al. Pediatric midface fractures: outcomes and complications of 218 patients. Laryngoscope Investig Otolaryngol 2019;4(6):597–601.

45. Pontell ME, Niklinska EB, Braun SA, et al. Resorbable versus titanium rigid fixation for pediatric mandibular fractures: a systematic review, institutional experience and comparative analysis. Craniomaxillofac Trauma Reconstr 2022;15(3):189–200.

46. Pontell ME, Niklinska EB, Braun SA, et al. Resorbable versus titanium hardware for rigid fixation of pediatric upper and midfacial fractures: which carries a lower risk profile? J Oral Maxillofac Surg 2021;79(10):2103–14.

47. An J, Jia P, Zhang Y, et al. Application of biodegradable plates for treating pediatric mandibular fractures. J Cranio-Maxillo-Fac Surg 2015;43(4):515–20.

48. Stone ME Jr, Farber BA, Olorunfemi O, et al. Penetrating neck trauma in children: an uncommon entity described using the National Trauma Data Bank. J Trauma Acute Care Surg 2016;80(4):604–9.

49. Li H, Li Z, Zhao J, et al. Management of paediatric laryngotracheal trauma. J Laryngol Otol 2022;136(11):1125–9.

50. Tessler RA, Nguyen H, Newton C, et al. Pediatric penetrating neck trauma: hard signs of injury and selective neck exploration. J Trauma Acute Care Surg 2017; 82(6):989–94.

51. Abdelmasih M, Kayssi A, Roche-Nagle G. Penetrating paediatric neck trauma. BMJ Case Rep 2019;12(5):e226436.

52. Carratola M, Hart CK. Pediatric tracheal trauma. Semin Pediatr Surg 2021;30(3): 151057.

Head & Neck Trauma in the Geriatric Population

Lucy L. Shi, MD[a], Jacey Pudney, MD[b], Sharon Brangman, MD[b],
Kourosh Parham, MD[c], Michael Nuara, MD[a],*

KEYWORDS

- Geriatrics • Elderly • Trauma • Maxillofacial • Facial fracture

KEY POINTS

- The incidence of geriatric maxillofacial trauma is likely to continue to rise with the aging population and have more unique presentations including a predominance of women, a higher proportion of midface fractures, and more frequently a result of falls.
- Multiple comorbidities and medical fragility in this population result in higher lengths of stay and mortality. Therefore, many medical considerations must be taken into account including preoperative risk assessment, capacity and functional evaluations, syncopal workups, and delirium prevention.
- Surgical technique may also differ in the geriatric population due to decreased bone stock, osteoporosis, and poor bony vascularity. In addition, goals such as aesthetics may be of lesser importance in this population.
- Quality improvement measures have been undertaken to help standardize the care for this vulnerable population.

INTRODUCTION

According to an estimation by the United Nations Department of Economic and Social Affairs, 20% of the world's population will be older than 65 years by 2050.[1] Similar trends have been predicted by the United States Census Bureau, demonstrating that by the year 2035, the population of adults older than 65 will outnumber children under the age of 18. Adults over the age of 85 is currently the fastest growing segment of the population.[2] Similarly, rates of geriatric trauma have also increased and these trends are expected to continue with a progressively aging demographic.[3,4]

Trauma is a common cause for emergency department presentation and hospitalization in the geriatric population. A number of factors including increased debilitation,

[a] Division of Facial Plastic & Reconstructive Surgery, Virginia Mason Franciscan Health, 1201 Terry Avenue 9th Floor, Seattle, WA 98101, USA; [b] Department of Geriatrics, SUNY Upstate University Hospital, 750 East Adams Street, Syracuse, NY 13210, USA; [c] Department of Otolaryngology–Head & Neck Surgery, University of Connecticut, 263 Farmington Avenue, Farmington, CT 06030, USA
* Corresponding author. 1201 Terry Avenue, Floor 9, Seattle, WA 98101.
E-mail address: michael.nuara@vmfh.org

Otolaryngol Clin N Am 56 (2023) 1183–1201
https://doi.org/10.1016/j.otc.2023.05.005
0030-6665/23/© 2023 Elsevier Inc. All rights reserved.
oto.theclinics.com

syncopal risk due to cardiovascular or neurologic comorbidities, and vision changes place older patients at higher risk of falls and other traumatic events.[5] In addition, as a growing segment of the geriatric population maintain their social lives and physical activity, the etiology of trauma will continue to evolve.[6] To date, maxillofacial trauma in the geriatric population has not been well-characterized. The purpose of this article is to better describe the presentation, perioperative management, surgical technique, and other considerations with relation to maxillofacial trauma in the elderly.

Epidemiology and Presentation

The incidence of trauma in the elderly, including fractures of the maxillofacial skeleton, has increased steadily over recent years.[3,4] From 2005 to 2015, the National Trauma Database (NTDB) reported an increase of geriatric trauma from 18% of all trauma to 30%.[7] Trauma in the elderly is associated with significantly worse outcomes compared to in younger populations. The elderly are more likely to be hospitalized, have longer length of stay (LOS), and have higher rates of unplanned ICU admissions.[8,9] In addition, delays in the surgical management of facial injuries were also noted to occur more frequently in the elderly population, likely due to the need for the perioperative stabilization of other comorbidities.[10] Trauma in the geriatric population has repeatedly been shown to be associated with higher rates of mortality, both during the immediate admission as well as in a delayed fashion.[11,12] For these reasons, elderly trauma patients face a much more arduous recovery course compared to younger cohorts.

The demographics and etiology of maxillofacial trauma in the elderly are different than that of younger populations. Facial fractures have traditionally been considered an affliction of young men but, in the geriatric population, most reports demonstrate a predominance of women.[13–17] This predominance has been noted to increase with age. This finding has been attributed to many factors. For one, while falls are considered the most common mechanism of injury in geriatric populations, older women are significantly more susceptible to falls than men.[13,18–20] Higher rates of osteoporosis amongst women have also been implicated as a cause for the higher rates of facial fracture.[15,21] Finally, women tend to have longer average lifespans compared to men, which may explain the higher rates of facial fractures amongst females with advancing age.[13] On the other hand, men were more likely to sustain injury as a result of sporting activities, motor vehicle accidents (MVAs), or assault.[6,19,22,23] Assault, unfortunately, remains prevalent even in the elderly and these victims were more likely to have severe trauma, require ICU admission, and have alcohol or drugs involved.[24,25]

In the United States, fractures of the midface and orbit were the most common sites of injury in the geriatric population (**Fig. 1**). These include zygomaticomaxillary complex (ZMC), orbital, and nasal bone fractures.[9,14,26,27] Globally, the data was more variable; most European studies also identified the midface as the most common site of fracture[20,28] while studies from Japan, China, and Nigeria reported the lower face to be the most common.[18,29,30] These differences may be a result of lifestyle, vehicle use, and a comparatively younger geriatric population in the non-Western countries. Fractures in the elderly have traditionally been associated with falls, but edentulousness, periodontitis, and osteoporosis likely also play a role in weakening the facial buttresses.[15,21] Mandibular fractures were typically described as the second most common site of facial fracture. Amongst geriatric patients with mandible fractures, condylar fractures were the most common subsite.[20,27] The presence of healthy teeth or third molars have been shown to impact the subsite where fractures occur by

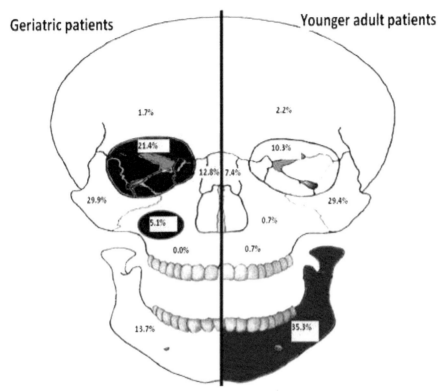

Fig. 1. Comparison of where fractures occur in the geriatric population. (Source: Toivari M, Helenius M, Suominen AL, Lindqvist C, Thoren H. Etiology of facial fractures in elderly Finns during 2006-2007. *Oral Surgery Oral Medicine Oral Pathology Oral Radiology.* Nov 2014;118(5):539-545.)

displacing the force.[31] It should also be noted that in the atrophic jaw, the placement of dental implants pose a risk for causing iatrogenic fracture.[32,33]

Geriatric facial trauma patients are significantly more likely to also have concurrent associated injuries compared to younger populations.[34–36] The most common concomitant injuries were those of the long bones, which were typically associated with MVAs.[30,34] Concurrent neurologic injuries, including cervical spine injuries and intracranial hemorrhages, were also significantly higher in the geriatric population.[30,37] In one report, brain injuries were fivefold more common in the elderly population.[38] Another report demonstrated a higher risk of ischemic stroke in elderly patients who sustained facial fractures.[39] As a large proportion of elderly patients are on anticoagulation, intracranial hemorrhage, and retro-orbital hematomas occur with higher frequencies as well.[40,41] A comprehensive trauma survey must therefore be completed on all geriatric trauma patients due to the high risk of associated injuries. A low threshold for trauma team activation and close observation should be employed.

Medical Considerations

Older adults have a higher prevalence of comorbidities which adds to the complexity of managing their perioperative care. Approximately 85% of patients over the age of 65 have one chronic disease and 60% have at least 2 or more including arthritis, hypertension, heart disease, diabetes, respiratory diseases, stroke, and cancer.[42] Within the geriatric facial trauma population, most reports describe the majority of patients having at least one comorbidity, with hypertension and cardiac problems being the most common.[13,19,20]

Medical Risk Assessment and Optimization

Many considerations exist when deciding to proceed with surgery in the geriatric population including physiologic comorbidities, functional status, anticoagulation, polypharmacy, and goals of care. To better define inappropriate medication prescription and limit polypharmacy in the elderly population, the American Geriatric Society (AGS) has developed the Beers© Criteria.[43] **Table 1** outlines important recommendations that should be addressed before surgery in older adults.

About 25% to 30% of postoperative deaths are from cardiac causes and are directly related to age.[44] For non-cardiac surgeries it is recommended to evaluate the patient's cardiovascular risk for surgery which may be classified as either mild risk (endoscopic procedures, superficial procedures, cataract surgery), intermediate risk (head and neck, intraperitoneal and intrathoracic, cardiac endarterectomy, orthopedic) or severe/vascular risk (aortic/other major vascular surgery). The preoperative cardiac assessment published by the American College of Cardiology and American Heart Association (ACC/AHA) provides a good algorithm for determining these risks (**Fig. 2**). **Table 2** presents a list of preoperative testing modalities and their indications.[43]

The presence of comorbidities has been shown to impact postoperative outcomes. One report found the presence of more than one comorbidity to be an independent predictor of death in their geriatric facial trauma population.[45] Another similar study identified ICU admission, acute renal failure, history of myocardial infarction, and coagulopathy as significantly increasing the odds ratio for mortality.[46] In an analysis of geriatric orthopedic trauma, the authors identified comorbidities such as diabetes to be more impactful on complication rate than osteoporosis or low bone quality.[47] As such, surgical risk assessment and medical optimization has important implications on surgical outcomes.

Cognitive and Functional Assessment

The initial preoperative assessment should include the patient's overall goals and expectations for surgery which are important for making an informed decision.[44]

The AGS recommends obtaining a baseline cognitive assessment before surgery. Patients with mild cognitive impairment and dementia are at higher risk for delirium and poorer postoperative outcomes.[44] Patients with cognitive impairment may need extra time to understand the procedure or provide consent. A healthcare proxy may be needed. The Mini-Cog© is a simple way to screen for dementia and consists of a three-item recall and clock drawing test with a maximum score of five.[48] Ask the patient to repeat three unrelated words (eg, banana, sunrise, chair) and tell them to remember these words to be asked later, with up to three tries. Next, have them draw a clock with the hands indicating a specific time; the clock must include all 12 numbers and the two hands must be in the appropriate place. A normal clock gives 2 points and each word recalled without prompting gives one point. A total Mini-Cog© score of 0 to 2 indicates a positive screen for dementia and a score of 3 to 5 is a negative screen.

Frailty and impaired physical function are associated with postoperative complications.[49] Frailty has also been associated with increased risk of discharge to a facility rather than home, higher rates of delirium, functional decline, and death.[44] To assess frailty, the FRAIL Scale can be used (**Table 3**).[50] The Katz Assessment for Activities of

	Rationale/Recommendations	Implementation
Table 1		
Preoperative recommendations for older adults		
Goals of care	Discuss patient's goals of care; what matters most to the patient.	Discussion with patients about risks, benefits, and quality of life.
Cognition	Evaluate patient's cognitive ability and capacity to understand the anticipated surgery and risks. Include both patient and family.	• Brief dementia screening • Administer Mini-Cog C
Functional status	Patients with impaired physical function are at risk for poor outcomes after surgery. Ask patient and family.	• Katz Index for Activities of Daily Living • Lawton Instrumental Activities of Daily Living
Frailty	Frailty is associated with: • Postoperative complications (POC) • Longer hospital stays • Higher rates of delirium • Functional decline	• FRAIL Scale • If frailty is present, use for risk stratification
Nutritional status	Poor nutritional status increases risk of post operative complications (POC)	Perioperative nutrition screen (PONS) • Assess BMI< 18.5 kg/m^2 • Weight loss of >10 lbs. in the last 6 mo • Reduced oral intake by >50% in the last week • Or preoperative serum albumin <3.0 g/dL If yes to any question should undergo preoperative nutrition evaluation
Cardiovascular risk	Risk of postoperative cardiac events is related to age. Perform preoperative cardiac evaluations.	• Estimate functional capacity in terms of metabolic equivalents • ACC/AHA algorithm • ASA classification
Pulmonary risk	Evaluate patient-related (age, COPD, ASA Class I or greater, heart failure) and procedure-related risks (emergency surgery, prolonged surgery, AAA repair, neurosurgery)	American College of Physicians Guideline for Risk Assessment and perioperative management of pulmonary complications
Kidney function	Renal and glomerular blood flow decrease with age	• Assess renal function, and adjust medications as needed
Medications	Increased risk for polypharmacy and risk of adverse drug reactions	• List for high-risk medication • Beers Criteria® (m) • Consider pharmacy consult. • Discuss with PCP for more complex medication review.
Anticoagulation	Similar to recommendations in younger adults	• Cessation of warfarin with or without low molecular-weight heparin bridge therapy based on risk of thromboembolism

(continued on next page)

Table 1 (continued)		
	Rationale/Recommendations	**Implementation**
		• Stop apixaban, rivaroxaban, and dabigatran 2–3 d before surgery depending on bleeding risk associated with the procedure.
Anesthesia Method	Insufficient evidence to recommend one anesthetic plan for all older adults	Adjust medications to renal and hepatic functions as needed

Daily Living (ADLs) measures activities including bathing, dressing, feeding, transferring, toileting, and continence (**Fig. 3**).[51] Patients with deficits in ADLs are at higher risk for postoperative complications.

A large proportion of geriatric trauma is caused by falls, which may belie other underlying deficits. A survey study on aging conducted in the UK identified chronic diseases, incontinence, depressive symptoms, and frailty as increasing the risk of falls.[5] A full workup should therefore be considered prior to discharge to evaluate these multifactorial etiologies.[52] A European group described a novel multidisciplinary pathway for syncopal workup comprising of tests for visual acuity, malnutrition, cognition, and consultation with a physical therapist. Cardiac testing, comprising of labs, orthostatic evaluation, and electrocardiogram (ECG) was then completed followed by neurologic testing with brain imaging and electroencephalogram (EEG) if needed.[53]

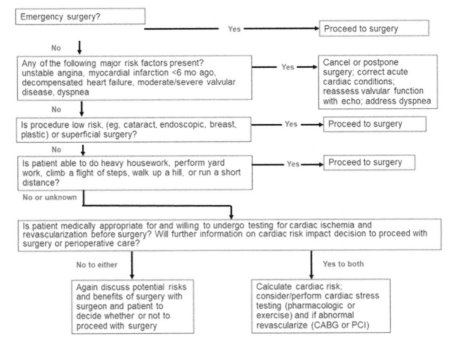

Fig. 2. American College of Cardiology and American Heart Association (ACC/AHA) preoperative cardiac risk assessment algorithm. (Reuben DB, Herr KA, Pacala JT, et al, *Geriatrics at your fingertips*, 23rd ed. American Geriatrics Society 2021:286.)

Table 2
Cardiac and pulmonary preoperative testing recommendations

Tests	Indication

Chest Radiograph (CXR)	• Not recommended for routine preoperative screening
	• Recommended for patients:
	  ○ Acute cardiopulmonary disease (by history or suspected on exam)
	  ○ Age >70 with history of stable chronic cardiopulmonary disease without CXR in past 6 mo
	  ○ Undergoing major surgical operation

Electrocardiogram (ECG)	• Not recommended for routine preoperative screening
	• Recommended for patients:
	  ○ Undergoing intermediate risk or vascular surgery
	  ○ With known ischemic heart disease, previous myocardial infarction, cardiac arrhythmia, peripheral vascular disease cerebrovascular disease, compensated or prior heart failure, diabetes, chronic kidney, or respiratory disease

Pulmonary Function Test (PFT)	• Not recommended for routine preoperative screening • Recommended for patients undergoing lung resections, thoracic surgery
Noninvasive Stress Testing	• Not recommended for routine preoperative screening, specifically in patients undergoing intermediate risk operation with no clinical risk factors and patients undergoing low risk operations • Reasonable for patients with 3 or more clinical risk factors and poor functional capacity undergoing vascular surgery. • Patients with at least one or two clinical risk factors and poor functional capacity who require intermediate risk or vascular surgery

Surgical Considerations

The rate of conservative versus surgical management was varied widely across studies. In general, fractures in the elderly were more likely to be treated conservatively compared to in younger patients.[15,18] The rate of surgical management declined with increasing age.[10,22,54] These findings may be a reflection of many factors, including the larger proportion of midface fractures in this cohort which are more often treated with observation, differing goals and less concerns for cosmesis, increased anesthetic risk, and preexisting functional deficits that obviate the benefits of repair.

In the following paragraphs, we will provide an overview of the specific technical considerations for geriatric maxillofacial fractures in each anatomic subsite.

Table 3
FRAIL scale

Fatigue	Do you feel fatigued?
Resistance	Can you walk up one flight of stairs without assistance?
Ambulation	Are you able to walk a few blocks without assistance or aids?
Illnesses	Do you have more than 5 illnesses?
Loss of weight	Have you lost 5% or more of your body weight in the last year?
Score: Robust (score 0), Prefrail (score 1–2), Frail (score 3–5)	

Patient Name:_____   Date:_____
Patient ID #_____

Katz Index of Independence in Activities of Daily Living

Activities Points (1 or 0)	Independence (1 Point)	Dependence (0 Points)
	NO supervision, direction or personal assistance.	WITH supervision, direction, personal assistance or total care.
BATHING Points: _____	(1 POINT) Bathes self completely or needs help in bathing only a single part of the body such as the back, genital area or disabled extremity.	(0 POINTS) Need help with bathing more than one part of the body, getting in or out of the tub or shower. Requires total bathing
DRESSING Points: _____	(1 POINT) Get clothes from closets and drawers and puts on clothes and outer garments complete with fasteners. May have help tying shoes.	(0 POINTS) Needs help with dressing self or needs to be completely dressed.
TOILETING Points: _____	(1 POINT) Goes to toilet, gets on and off, arranges clothes, cleans genital area without help.	(0 POINTS) Needs help transferring to the toilet, cleaning self or uses bedpan or commode.
TRANSFERRING Points: _____	(1 POINT) Moves in and out of bed or chair unassisted. Mechanical transfer aids are acceptable	(0 POINTS) Needs help in moving from bed to chair or requires a complete transfer.
CONTINENCE Points:	(1 POINT) Exercises complete self control over urination and defecation.	(0 POINTS) Is partially or totally incontinent of bowel or bladder
FEEDING Points: _____	(1 POINT) Gets food from plate into mouth without help. Preparation of food may be done by another person.	(0 POINTS) Needs partial or total help with feeding or requires parenteral feeding.

TOTAL POINTS: _____   SCORING: 6 = High (*patient independent*) 0 = Low (*patient very dependent*

Source:
try this: Best Practices in Nursing Care to Older Adults, The Hartford Institute for Geriatric Nursing, New York University, College of Nursing, www.hartfordign.org.

MaineHealth

Fig. 3. Katz index of independence in activities of daily living.

Lower Face

Cephalometric studies using radiographic imaging have demonstrated significantly decreased mandibular ramus height, body height, and body length with age.[55] To better describe mandibular atrophy, Luhr and colleagues created a classification system based on body height with class I being 16 to 20 mm, class II being 11 to 15 mm, and class 3 being $\leq$10 mm.[56] Management of fractures in the edentulous atrophic mandible remains an area of continuous debate.

The treatment of mandible fractures has undergone significant change over time. Prior to the mid-1900s, the fractured atrophic mandible was generally treated nonoperatively or with closed reduction using maxillomandibular fixation (MMF). Gunning splints, developed by Thomas Gunning in 1863, were casts created from impressions taken of the patient's mandible and maxilla and used as an intra-oral cast for the fractured mandible. As dentures have become more commonly available, a variety of closed fixation methods were developed including circumandibular wiring of the patient's dentures across a mandibular fracture, circumzygomatic or pyriform aperture wiring to stabilize the fracture using an upper denture, and circumandibular wiring directly across the fracture itself. Finally, a severely comminuted fracture or a fracture with significant soft tissue damage could be treated through external fixation.[57] In patients with significant comorbidities that preclude surgery, closed reduction is a viable option to stabilize the fracture while avoiding other risks. However, many elderly patients have difficulty tolerating prolonged periods in MMF and the risk of nonunion is more common.[58,59]

Open reduction with internal fixation (ORIF) allows for direct exposure and fixation of the fracture. The approach can be either transcutaneous or transoral approach. In the elderly, a supraperiosteal dissection is advocated by some surgeons to preserve the vascular supply to the bone.[57,58] The AO Foundation (Arbeitsgemeinschaft für Osteosynthesefragen) currently recommends ORIF with the use of a locking 2.4 mm reconstruction plate.[59] A large load-bearing plate with bicortical screws is more likely to withstand masticatory forces, limit the risk of hardware breakage, and allow for immediate return to function.[60–63] At least three screws are recommended to be placed in each fracture segment, ideally in the symphysis and angle regions where the bone stock is best.[59,64] Criticisms of a large compression plate include the higher risk of causing a fracture by screw placement, compromised healing due to wider dissection, potential for inferior alveolar nerve damage with consequent lip hypoesthesia, and plate extrusion.[57,65] Studies have suggested similar union rates and complications between two miniplates and large reconstruction plates, but these authors still recommend decision-making be made on a case by case basis.[66,67] The advent of the 2.0 mm load-bearing plate has allowed for a lower profile plate with load-bearing properties.[58] In general, most surgeons feel the smaller the mandible, the more important it is to rigidly fixate with a larger caliber plate to account for the greater amount of masticatory force per unit area of bone. This may not be as important in a patient who is already on a mechanical soft diet for unrelated reasons.

Condylar or subcondylar fractures of the edentulous mandible represent a unique situation that, unlike in the dentate patient, cannot be easily treated with closed reduction and MMF. Open reduction remains the recommended treatment.[68,69] Close observation with the use of ORIF only when loss of ramus height presents is one option.[70] Combined use of a patient's dentures or Gunning splint with carefully placed MMF screws is another option.[71]

New technologies have arisen in recent years to aid in the management of these complex fractures. Augmentation of the fractured mandible is sometimes necessary to aid in bone healing and address continuity defects and anterior iliac crest bone has historically been the most common donor site.[58,59] To avoid donor site morbidity, various allogenic materials have been described including bone cement, a resorbable mesh system, and bone morphogenetic proteins.[72–75] In select cases, a vascularized free bone flap has been used with good outcomes.[76,77] The use of virtual surgical planning (VSP) to create custom-bent plates has also been employed, demonstrating good outcomes in bone union and decreased operative time.[78–80] In light of the medical fragility of these patients, techniques to decrease anesthetic time and surgical sites can reduce overall morbidity.

Midface

Fractures of the midface, including of the zygoma, the maxilla, and the nasal bones, are the most common site of geriatric facial fractures.[9,18] The mechanism of falls and higher rates of osteoporosis have been implicated in these findings.[21,81] Periodontitis and edentulousness have also been shown to increase the risk of osteoporosis and facial fractures.[82] These factors likely play a role in yielding more unusual fracture patterns within this population.

There is a paucity of literature on the surgical management of these injuries. In general, the management of midface fractures varies greatly. The primary indication for ORIF in this area is to maintain the aesthetic projection and height of the face. Rarely, impingement of the muscles of mastication or coronoid process with subsequent trismus may also occur.[83] Delayed presentation of lower eyelid ectropion from depressed malar fracture is an underreported sequela that should also be monitored. Given the medical fragility of these patients, a conservative approach is more likely to be undertaken when the objective is aesthetics.[84] When surgical management is undertaken, standard midface techniques with closed reduction or miniplate fixation is appropriate in this population as well.[84,85] The placement of alloplastic facial implants have been described for facial augmentation in the atrophic posttraumatic midface.[86] In our experience, function is typically prioritized far more than cosmesis and patients more often will choose an observational approach when function is minimally impacted.

Orbit

Orbital fractures occur more commonly in the elderly and have a higher chance of being severe or extensive, with an area of 2 cm^2 or greater.[15,27,87] Of these, the orbital floor was the most common subsite of fracture.[9,21] The rate of ocular injuries and retroorbital hematomas, secondary to anticoagulation use, is also higher in this population.[41,87]

Generally, practitioners are more reluctant to operate on orbital fractures in this population. In one single-institution review of 25 geriatric orbital fractures, only two were managed surgically, one for persistent diplopia and the other due to defect size.[88] Postsurgical complications may be more common in geriatric patients managed surgically, including lower eyelid malposition.[89] On the other hand, it is important to note that untreated visual disturbances in this population can be very impactful and increase the risk of future injuries.[22] In a recent quality of life survey study, peripheral vision and vision specific roles were the only measures found to have declined following facial trauma in the geriatric population.[90] We strongly emphasize the importance of repeated follow-up ophthalmological evaluation in all cases, regardless of initial fracture management.

Postoperative Care and Follow-up

Geriatric trauma patients typically experience a more extended LOS compared to younger cohorts.[9,34] Some surgeons may opt to perform early postoperative imaging depending on the complexity of the case. **Table 4** describes recommendations for the medical management of postoperative geriatric patients.

Delirium is one of the major complications in hospitalized older adults and can occur in 30% to 40% of post-operative patients. Delirium is associated with increased medical costs, increased LOS, and increase in 1-year mortality.[49] The Confusion Assessment Method (**Table 5**) is a useful tool to evaluate a patient for delirium. **Table 6** describes a list of factors that may increase its risk.

Depending on the choice of internal fixation and surgeon discretion, patients can return to a liquid or semi-liquid diet postoperatively. Maintenance of oral hygiene, including avoidance of alcohol and tobacco, remains imperative during the immediate postoperative course. Chlorhexidine oral rinses (0.12%), or with a combination of 3%

Table 4
Postoperative recommendations for older adults

	Concern	Intervention
Pain	• Older adults and those with cognitive impairment are at high risk for undertreated pain • Inadequate pain control increases risk for delirium • Use multi-system approach	• Scheduled acetaminophen (if applicable, max of 3 g daily) • Topical options (diclofenac gel/lidocaine patches) • Opioids: Lowest effective dose for shortest time • Avoid NSAIDs: risk for GI bleeding, delirium, fluid retention, nephrotoxicity, CVS risks • Avoid muscle relaxants due to increased risk of delirium
Delirium	• Delirium is linked to POC and poor outcomes • Assess for delirium and try to reduce risk factors • Can use CAM Score to assess for delirium	• Nonpharmacological delirium precaution to reduce risk: ○ Reduce sleep interruption ○ Avoid dehydration ○ Encourage mobility, avoid restraints and IV's when able ○ Enhance sensory input (make sure patients have eyeglasses, hearing aids, dentures) ○ Minimize anticholinergic medications ○ Control pain, constipation ○ Correct abnormal electrolytes
GI concerns	High risk for constipation and diarrhea	• Scheduled laxatives when prescribing opioids • For diarrhea, check for fecal impaction, ○ If on antibiotics, consider check for leukocytes or *Clostridium difficile*
Kidney function	Watch for early signs of acute kidney injury: oliguria, isosthenuria, increase in serum creatinine	• Hold nephrotoxic medications • If GU obstruction, insert bladder catheter
Urinary	Older patients have a higher prevalence of voiding dysfunction; especially men with prostate hyperplasia	• Monitor urinary output • Limit anticholinergic medication • Constipation can contribute to urinary retention

hydrogen peroxide for more significant debris, is generally prescribed at least three times a day postoperatively. Follow up is recommended 1 week postoperatively to assess for infection and fracture stability with close examination thereafter at the surgeon's discretion.[59]

Geriatric patients are more likely to require healthcare resources upon discharge, including inpatient rehabilitation or chronic care facility use.[9] Patients discharged to these facilities were also found to have higher rates of mortality at 1-year compared to patients discharged to home.[12] Elder neglect and abuse must be considered as well, which can manifest physically as well as emotionally and financially, and occurs more frequently amongst minority groups, females, and patients with dementia or

Table 5
Confusion assessment method (CAM)

Criteria	Evidence
1. Acute change in mental status	Observation by family/caregiver, RN, MD
2. Symptoms that fluctuate over minutes or hours	Observation by nursing staff or caregiver
3. Inattention	Patient history, poor digit recall, inability or recite months backwards
4. Altered level of consciousness	Hyper alertness, drowsiness, stupor or coma
5. Disorganized thinking	Rambling or incoherent speech, irrelevant conversation or an unclear or illogical flow of ideas

- The first 3 criteria plus either the 4th or 5th criteria must be present to confirm a diagnosis of delirium
- For patients with known psychiatric disease, disorganized thinking may be present at baseline, so all 5 criteria must be present to diagnose delirium.

Adapted from Inouye S, Annals of Internal Medicine; 1990; 113: 941–948.

functional disability.[91,92] When evaluating the older adult for discharge, clinicians may feel pressure to discharge to a care facility, sometimes contradicting the patient's wishes. A multidisciplinary team with the careful evaluation of capacity can be beneficial in making these decisions.[93]

Quality Improvement

Geriatric maxillofacial trauma is at the intersection of two quality improvement initiatives of the American College of Surgeons (ACS)/AGS Trauma Quality Improvement Program (TQIP).[94] TQIP collects data from nearly 900 trauma centers and provides best practice guidelines for managing various patient populations. In 2013, it published a geriatric trauma management guideline (Link 1), and in a separate guideline last revised in 2019 (Link 2), addresses elder abuse as a part of guidelines to recognize child, elder, and intimate partner violence. The 2013 geriatric trauma guidelines emphasized the importance of specialized geriatric inpatient care, ongoing assessment of capacity, and documentation of care preferences.[43]

Development of elderly-specific care protocols within the multidisciplinary trauma service model is essential to reducing mortality and morbidity in this population through better risk assessment, adherence to preventive strategies, and timely recognition of complications. Key recommendations include.

- Lower threshold for the activation of the trauma team. Trivial mechanisms which in the elderly could cause more significant injury and preexisting conditions which could blunt the physiological response to injury can result in the late recognition of life-threatening injury.
- Recognize the presence of comorbidities and polypharmacy. The secondary survey should therefore also emphasize the accurate documentation of medications.
- Evaluate for injury with imaging when appropriate as trivial mechanisms may lead to serious injury in this vulnerable population.
- Assessment of the use of anticoagulation, which can lead to higher risk of hemorrhage. Coagulation labs can be helpful and rapid reversal of anticoagulation, when possible, has been associated with improved outcomes after injury.

Table 6
Delirium risk factors and recommendations for prevention or intervention

Risks Factors	Interventions
Age ≥ 70	Unmodifiable
Cognitive impairment	• Write day of week/date, names of staff on whiteboard in room • Orient patient to day and night • Assist with food trays and feeding if needed. • Allow family members to stay with patient when possible • Uninterrupted sleep (avoid overnight room changes, unnecessary blood draws/tests, vital checks, or medications overnight) • Monitor for pain (may need to use nonverbal assessment tools in some patients)
Decreased sensory input	• Ensure patient has eyeglasses, hearing aids, dentures
History of alcohol abuse	• Screen for withdrawal
Limited physical functioning	• Assess functional status and assist where needed (toileting, grooming, using telephone or other technology)
Undertreated pain	• Scheduled acetaminophen three times a day (no more than 3 g if no hepatic impairment). Avoid prn dosing. • Low dose short acting opioids • Lidocaine patch, diclofenac gel • Heating pads and ice packs
Inappropriate medications	• Use Beers Criteria® to reduce risk of adverse drug events (m) • Avoid anticholinergic medications when possible • Avoid NSAIDs, benzodiazepines, muscle relaxers
Abnormal serum sodium, potassium or glucose, low hemoglobin	• Monitor laboratories • Assess nutritional status and intake
Postoperative Immobility	• Physical therapy consultation • Out of bed as soon as possible
Constipation	• Scheduled bowel regimen • Monitor output
Urinary retention	• Monitor output; consider bladder scan if no urinary output
Medical emergencies such as myocardial infarctions or pulmonary embolisms	• Use appropriate venous thrombosis prophylaxis • Monitor laboratories and pain

In 2016, the ACS National Surgical Quality Improvement Program (NSQIP) published another geriatric-specific guideline. In 2019, ACS launched the Geriatric Surgery Verification (GSV) Program with 32 standards addressing elements such as administrative commitment, geriatric-friendly facilities, and establishing protocols for shared decision-making and transitions of care. Preliminary data have demonstrated reductions in LOS already with this new program.[95]

SUMMARY

Craniofacial trauma in the geriatric population is increasing as our population ages and can be very severe. Unique medical and surgical considerations must be taken into account in the management of this vulnerable population.

CLINICS CARE POINTS

- Geriatric maxillofacial trauma presents more uniquely compared to other age groups including a higher proportion of midface fractures, a predominance of women, and more frequently a result of falls.

- Due to the medical fragility in this population, meticulous preoperative risk assessment and testing should be undertaken before proceeding with surgery. Patients typically have higher lengths of stay and mortality.

- Falls are sometimes a sign of cognitive and functional decline, which can be worsened due to delirium and hospitalizations. These impairments should be taken into consideration for safe discharge planning.

- In fractures of the mandible, edentulousness and decreased bone stock must be taken into consideration when planning repair, and load-bearing plates are often used.

- Generally, midface and orbital fractures are managed conservatively in this population due to increased medical comorbidities and a lessened importance of aesthetic goals.

DISCLOSURES

None.

REFERENCES

1. Division P. World population ageing: 1950-2050. United Nations Publications Department of Economic and Social Affairs; 2002.
2. Vespa J. The US Joins Other Countries with Large Aging Populations. United States Census Bureau. https://www.census.gov/library/stories/2018/03/graying-america.html.
3. Baidwan NK, Naranje SM. Epidemiology and recent trends of geriatric fractures presenting to the emergency department for United States population from year 2004-2014. Publ Health 2017;142:64–9.
4. Bonne S, Schuerer DJE. Trauma in the Older Adult Epidemiology and Evolving Geriatric Trauma Principles. Clin Geriatr Med 2013;29(1):137–+.
5. Gale CR, Cooper C, Sayer AA. Prevalence and risk factors for falls in older men and women: The English Longitudinal Study of Ageing. Age Ageing 2016;45(6):789–94.
6. Plawecki A, Bobian M, Kandinov A, et al. Recreational Activity and Facial Trauma Among Older Adults. Jama Facial Plastic Surgery 2017;19(6):453–8.
7. Jiang LB, Zheng ZJ, Zhang M. The incidence of geriatric trauma is increasing and comparison of different scoring tools for the prediction of in-hospital mortality in geriatric trauma patients. World J Emerg Surg 2020;15(1):59.
8. Mulvey HE, Haslam RD, Laytin AD, et al. Unplanned ICU Admission Is Associated With Worse Clinical Outcomes in Geriatric Trauma Patients. J Surg Res 2020;245: 13–21.
9. Mundinger GS, Bellamy JL, Miller DT, et al. Defining Population-Specific Craniofacial Fracture Patterns and Resource Use in Geriatric Patients: A Comparative Study of Blunt Craniofacial Fractures in Geriatric versus Nongeriatric Adult Patients. Plast Reconstr Surg 2016;137(2):386E–93E.
10. Brucoli M, Boffano P, Romeo I, et al. Management of maxillofacial trauma in the elderly: A European multicenter study. Dent Traumatol 2020;36(3):241–6.
11. Callaway DW, Wolfe R. Geriatric trauma. Emerg Med Clin 2007;25(3):837–+.

12. Huntington CR, Kao AM, Sing RF, et al. Unseen Burden of Injury: Post-Hospitalization Mortality in Geriatric Trauma Patients. Am Surg 2021. https://doi.org/10.1177/00031348211046886. 00031348211046886.

13. Brucoli M, Boffano P, Romeo I, et al. Epidemiology of maxillofacial trauma in the elderly: A European multicenter study. J Stomatol Oral Maxillofac Surg 2020; 121(4):330–8.

14. Stanbouly D, Baron M, Chang J, et al. Geriatric Craniomaxillofacial Fractures: Where do They Happen and Why? J Oral Maxillofac Surg 2022;80(10):1655–62.

15. Irgebay Z, Kahan EH, Park KE, et al. Characteristics and Patterns of Facial Fractures in the Elderly Population in the United States Based on Trauma Quality Improvement Project Data. J Craniofac Surg Jul-Aug 2022;33(5):1294–8.

16. Brown CVR, Rix K, Klein AL, et al. A Comprehensive Investigation of Comorbidities, Mechanisms, Injury Patterns, and Outcomes in Geriatric Blunt Trauma Patients. Am Surg 2016;82(11):1055–62.

17. Moreland B, Kakara R, Henry A. Trends in Nonfatal Falls and Fall-Related Injuries Among Adults Aged >= 65 Years - United States, 2012-2018. Mmwr-Morbidity and Mortality Weekly Report 2020;69(27):875–81.

18. Bojino A, Roccia F, Carlaw K, et al. A multicentric prospective analysis of maxillofacial trauma in the elderly population. Dent Traumatol 2022;38(3):185–95.

19. Aytac I, Yazici A, Tunc O. Maxillofacial Trauma in Geriatric Population. J Craniofac Surg 2020;31(7):E695–8.

20. Burkhard JPM, Pitteloud C, Klukowska-Rötzler J, et al. Changing trends in epidemiology and management of facial trauma in a Swiss geriatric population. Gerodontology 2019;36(4):358–64.

21. Zelken JA, Khalifian S, Mundinger GS, et al. Defining Predictable Patterns of Craniomaxillofacial Injury in the Elderly: Analysis of 1,047 Patients. J Oral Maxillofac Surg 2014;72(2):352–61.

22. Diab J, Moore MH. Facial fractures in the elderly: epidemiology, clinical characteristics, and management. Eur J Plast Surg 2021;44(5):577–86.

23. Possebon APD, Faot GGF, Pinto LD, et al. Etiology, diagnosis, and demographic analysis of maxillofacial trauma in elderly persons: A 10-year investigation. J Cranio-Maxillofacial Surg 2017;45(12):1921–6.

24. Rosen T, Clark S, Bloemen EM, et al. Geriatric assault victims treated at US trauma centers: Five-year analysis of the national trauma data bank. Injury-International Journal of the Care of the Injured 2016;47(12):2671–8.

25. Cillo JE, Holmes TM. Interpersonal Violence Is Associated With Increased Severity of Geriatric Facial Trauma. J Oral Maxillofac Surg 2016;74(5). https://doi.org/10.1016/j.joms.2016.01.003.

26. Marchini L, Allareddy V. Epidemiology of facial fractures among older adults: A retrospective analysis of a nationwide emergency department database. Dent Traumatol 2019;35(2):109–14.

27. Gray E, Dierks E, Homer L, et al. Survey of trauma patients requiring maxillofacial intervention, ages 56 to 91 years, with length of stay analysis. J Oral Maxillofac Surg 2002;60(10):1114–25.

28. Toivari M, Helenius M, Suominen AL, et al. Etiology of facial fractures in elderly Finns during 2006-2007. Oral Surgery Oral Medicine Oral Pathology Oral Radiology 2014;118(5):539–45.

29. Ito R, Kubota K, Inui A, et al. Oral-maxillofacial trauma of a geriatric population in a super-ageing country. Dent Traumatol 2017;33(6):433–7.

30. Liu FC, Halsey JN, Oleck NC, et al. Facial Fractures as a Result of Falls in the Elderly: Concomitant Injuries and Management Strategies. Craniomaxillofacial Trauma Reconstr 2019;12(1):45–53.

31. Nogami S, Yamauchi K, Yamashita T, et al. Elderly patients with maxillofacial trauma: study of mandibular condyle fractures. Dent Traumatol 2015;31(1):73–6.

32. Steiner T, Holzle F, Deppe H, et al. Postimplantation fracture in atrophic mandibles: A literature review completed with a case report. Implantologie 2012; 20(2):227–31.

33. Soehardi A, Meijer GJ, Manders R, et al. An Inventory of Mandibular Fractures Associated with Implants in Atrophic Edentulous Mandibles: A Survey of Dutch Oral and Maxillofacial Surgeons. Int J Oral Maxillofac Implants Sep-Oct 2011; 26(5):1087–93.

34. Diab J, Flapper W, Grave B, et al. A comparative analysis of associated injuries in the elderly and youth for facial fractures. J Plast Reconstr Aesthetic Surg 2022; 75(6):1979–87.

35. Toivari M, Suominen AL, Lindqvist C, et al. Among Patients With Facial Fractures, Geriatric Patients Have an Increased Risk for Associated Injuries. J Oral Maxillofac Surg 2016;74(7):1403–9.

36. Kokko LL, Puolakkainen T, Suominen A, et al. Are the Elderly With Maxillofacial Injuries at Increased Risk of Associated Injuries? J Oral Maxillofac Surg 2022; 80(8):1354–60.

37. Jarab F, Bataineh A. Pattern of Facial Fractures and Its Association with a Cervical Spine Injury in a Tertiary Hospital in Jordan. Int J Clin Pract 2022. https://doi.org/10.1155/2022/4107382. 20224107382.

38. Toivari M, Snall J, Suominen AL, et al. Associated Injuries Are Frequent and Severe Among Geriatric Patients With Zygomatico-Orbital Fractures. J Oral Maxillofac Surg 2019;77(3):565–70.

39. Kim R, Kim J, Jun Y, et al. Risk of Ischemic Stroke After a Facial Bone Fracture in Elderly Patients. Ann Plast Surg 2019;82(2):169–73.

40. Shimoni Z, Danilov V, Hadar S, et al. Head Computed Tomography Scans in Elderly Patients with Low Velocity Head trauma after a Fall. Isr Med Assoc J 2021;23(6):359–63.

41. Maurer P, Conrad-Hengerer I, Hollstein S, et al. Orbital haemorrhage associated with orbital fractures in geriatric patients on antiplatelet or anticoagulant therapy. Int J Oral Maxillofac Surg 2013;42(12):1510–4.

42. Talking with Your Older Patients. NIH National Institute on Aging. https://www.nia.nih.gov/health/talking-your-older-patients.

43. Chow WB, Rosenthal RA, Merkow RP, et al. Optimal Preoperative Assessment of the Geriatric Surgical Patient: A Best Practices Guideline from the American College of Surgeons National Surgical Quality Improvement Program and the American Geriatrics Society. J Am Coll Surg 2012;215(4):453–66.

44. Harper G, Lyons W, Potter J. Geriatrics review syllabus: a core curriculum in geriatric medicine. 11th Edition. New York: American Geriatrics Society; 2022.

45. Patel N, Le TN, Demissie S, et al. Factors Predictive of Mortality among Geriatric Patients Sustaining Low-Energy Blunt Trauma. Healthcare 2022;10(11):2214.

46. Clavijo-Alvarez JA, Deleyiannis FWB, Peitzman AB, et al. Risk Factors for Death in Elderly Patients With Facial Fractures Secondary to Falls. J Craniofac Surg 2012; 23(2):494–8.

47. Chen YB, Han YD, Niu ZH, et al. Is Decreased Local Bone Quality an Independent Risk Factor for Complications Following Fracture Fixation of Facial Bones. J Craniofac Surg 2021;32(4):1385–90.

48. Borson S, Scanlan JM, Sadak T, et al. Dementia Services Mini-Screen: A Simple Method to Identify Patients and Caregivers in Need of Enhanced Dementia Care Services. Am J Geriatr Psychiatr 2014;22(8):746–55.
49. Dogrul RT, Dogrul AB, Konan A, et al. Does Preoperative Comprehensive Geriatric Assessment and Frailty Predict Postoperative Complications? World J Surg 2020;44(11):3729–36.
50. Gleason LJ, Benton EA, Alvarez-Nebreda ML, et al. FRAIL Questionnaire Screening Tool and Short-Term Outcomes in Geriatric Fracture Patients. J Am Med Dir Assoc 2017;18(12):1082–6.
51. Best Practices in Nursing Care to Older Adults. The Hartford Institute for Geriatric Nursing. www.hartfordign.org.
52. Grubb BP, Karabin B. Syncope Evaluation and Management in the Geriatric Patient. Clin Geriatr Med 2012;28(4):717–+.
53. Wold JFH, Ruiter JH, Cornel JH, et al. A multidisciplinary care pathway for the evaluation of falls and syncope in geriatric patients. European Geriatric Medicine 2015;6(5):487–94.
54. Imholz B, Combescure C, Scolozzi P. Is age of the patient an independent predictor influencing the management of cranio-maxillo-facial trauma? A retrospective study of 308 patients. Oral Surgery Oral Medicine Oral Pathology Oral Radiology 2014;117(6):690–6.
55. Shaw RB, Katzel EB, Koltz PF, et al. Aging of the Mandible and Its Aesthetic Implications. Plastic and Reconstructive Surgery 2010;125(1):332–42.
56. Luhr HG, Reidick T, Merten HA. Results of treatment of fractures of the atrophic edentulous mandible by compression plating: A retrospective evaluation of 84 consecutive cases. J Oral Maxillof Surg 1996;54(3):250–4.
57. Madsen MJ, Haug RH, Christensen BS, et al. Management of Atrophic Mandible Fractures. Oral Maxillofac Surg Clin 2009;21(2):175–+.
58. Ellis E, Price C. Treatment protocol for fractures of the atrophic mandible. J Oral Maxillofac Surg 2008;66(3):421–35.
59. Ellis EI, Schubert W. Fractures of the edentulous atrophic mandible. AO Surgery Reference. https://surgeryreference.aofoundation.org/cmf/trauma/mandible/further-reading/fractures-in-the-edentulous-atrophic-mandible.
60. Gerbino G, Cocis S, Roccia F, et al. Management of atrophic mandibular fractures: An Italian multicentric retrospective study. J Cranio-Maxillofacial Surg 2018;46(12):2176–81.
61. Muller S, Burgers R, Ehrenfeld M, et al. Macroplate fixation of fractures of the edentulous atrophic mandible: immediate function and masticatory rehabilitation. Clin Oral Invest 2011;15(2):151–6.
62. Madsen MJ, Kushner GM, Alpert B. Failed Fixation in Atrophic Mandibular Fractures: The Case against Miniplates. Craniomaxillofacial Trauma Reconstr 2011; 4(3):145–50.
63. Santos GS, Costa M, Costa CD, et al. Failure of Miniplate Osteosynthesis for the Management of Atrophic Mandibular Fracture. J Craniofac Surg 2013;24(4): E415–8.
64. Pereira VA, da Silva BN, Reis JMN, et al. Effect of the number of screws on the stability of locking mandibular reconstruction plates. Int J Oral Maxillofac Surg 2013;42(6):732–5.
65. Novelli G, Sconza C, Ardito E, et al. Surgical Treatment of the Atrophic Mandibular Fractures by Locked Plates Systems: Our Experience and a Literature Review. Craniomaxillofacial Trauma & Reconstruction 2012;5(2):65–74.

66. Seu M, Jazayeri HE, Lopez J, et al. Comparing Load-Sharing Miniplate and Load-Bearing Plate Fixation in Atrophic Edentulous Mandibular Fractures: A Systematic Review and Meta-Analysis. J Craniofac Surg 2021;32(7):2401–5.

67. Brucoli M, Boffano P, Romeo I, et al. Surgical management of unilateral body fractures of the edentulous atrophic mandible. Oral and Maxillofacial Surgery-Heidelberg 2020;24(1):65–71.

68. Zachariades N, Mezitis M, Mourouzis C, et al. Fractures of the mandibular condyle: A review of 466 cases. Literature review, reflections on treatment and proposals. J Cranio-Maxillofacial Surg 2006;34(7):421–32.

69. Laskin DM. Management of Condylar Process Fractures. Oral Maxillofac Surg Clin 2009;21(2):193.

70. Brucoli M, Boffano P, Romeo I, et al. Management of mandibular condylar fractures in patients with atrophic edentulous mandibles. J\ Stomatol Oral Maxillof Surg 2020;121(3):226–32.

71. Chaudhary Z, Sharma R, Krishnan S. Maxillo Mandibular Fixation in Edentulous Scenarios: Combined MMF Screws and Gunning Splints. J Maxillof Oral Surg 2014;13(2):213–4.

72. Wolff KD, Swaid S, Nolte D, et al. Degradable injectable bone cement in maxillofacial surgery: indications and clinical experience in 27 patients. J Cranio-Maxillof Surg 2004;32(2):71–9.

73. Louis P, Holmes J, Fernandes R. Resorbable mesh as a containment system in reconstruction of the atrophic mandible fracture. J Oral Maxillofac Surg 2004; 62(6):719–23.

74. Castro-Nunez J, Cunningham LL, Van Sickels JE. Atrophic Mandible Fractures: Are Bone Grafts Necessary? An Update. J Oral Maxillofac Surg 2017;75(11): 2391–8.

75. Del Barrio RAL, de Souza ER, Al Houch AO, et al. Rehabilitation of Severely Atrophic Mandible: A 3-Year Follow-Up Protocol. J Oral Implantol 2022;48(6):475–9.

76. Zide MF, Ducic Y. Fibula microvascular free tissue reconstruction of the severely comminuted atrophic mandible fracture - case report. J Cranio-Maxillofacial Surg 2003;31(5):296–8.

77. De Feudis F, De Benedittis M, Antonicelli V, et al. Decision-making algorithm in treatment of the atrophic mandible fractures. Giornale Di Chirurgia Mar-Apr 2014;35(3–4):94–100.

78. Abbate V, Committeri U, Troise S, et al. Virtual Surgical Reduction in Atrophic Edentulous Mandible Fractures: A Novel Approach Based on "in House" Digital Work-Flow. Applied Sciences-Basel 2023;13(3):1474.

79. Castro-Nunez J, Shelton JM, Snyder S, et al. Virtual Surgical Planning for the Management of Severe Atrophic Mandible Fractures. Craniomaxillofacial Trauma Reconstr 2018;11(2):150–6.

80. Onodera K, Ohashi Y, Tsunoda N, et al. Computer-assisted surgery to treat fracture of an atrophic mandible. J Oral Maxillof Surg Med Pathol 2020;32(4):303–6.

81. Werning JW, Downey NM, Brinker RA, et al. The impact of osteoporosis on patients with maxillofacial trauma. Arch Otolaryngol Head Neck Surg 2004;130(3): 353–6.

82. Hong SJ, Yang BE, Yoo DM, et al. Analysis of the relationship between periodontitis and osteoporosis/fractures: a cross-sectional study. Bmc Oral Health 2021; 21(1):125.

83. Homsi N, Paulo R, Aniceto G, Hammer B, Bartlett S. Examination of patients with mid-facial fractures. AO Surgery Reference. https://surgeryreference.aofoundation.org/cmf/trauma/midface/further-reading/examination-of-patients-with-midfacial-injuries.

84. Cortese A, Caggiano M, Carlino F, et al. Zygomatic fractures: Technical modifications for better aesthetic and functional results in older patients. Int J Surg 2016; 33:S9–15.

85. Hohlweg-Majert B, Schmelzeisen R, Pfeiffer BM, et al. Significance of osteoporosis in craniomaxillofacial surgery: A review of the literature. Osteoporosis International 2006;17(2):167–79.

86. Matros E, Momoh A, Yaremchuk MJ. The Aging Midfacial Skeleton: Implications for Rejuvenation and Reconstruction Using Implants. Facial Plast Surg 2009; 25(4):252–9.

87. Toivari M, Suominen AL, Apajalahti S, et al. Isolated Orbital Fractures Are Severe Among Geriatric Patients. J Oral Maxillofac Surg 2018;76(2):388–95.

88. Patel AU, Haas JA, Skibba KE, et al. Outcomes Following Orbital Floor Fractures in the Elderly. J Craniofac Surg Jul-Aug 2020;31(5):1376–8.

89. Rajantie H, Nikunen M, Raj R, et al. Ageing increases risk of lower eyelid malposition after primary orbital fracture reconstruction. Br J Oral Maxillofac Surg 2022; 60(10):1391–6.

90. Boffano P, Pau A, Dosio C, et al. Quality of life following maxillofacial trauma in the elderly: a multicenter, prospective study. Oral and Maxillofacial Surgery-Heidelberg 2022;26(3):383–92.

91. Rosen T, Elman A, Clark S, et al. Vulnerable Elder Protection Team: Initial experience of an emergency department-based interdisciplinary elder abuse program. J Am Geriatr Soc 2022;70(11):3260–72.

92. Wong SP, Sharda N, Zietlow KE, et al. Planning for a Safe Discharge: More Than a Capacity Evaluation. J Am Geriatr Soc 2020;68(4):859–66.

93. El-Qawaqzeh K, Hosseinpour H, Gries L, et al. Dealing with the elder abuse epidemic: Disparities in interventions against elder abuse in trauma centers. J Am Geriatr Soc 2023. https://doi.org/10.1111/jgs.18286.

94. Nathens AB, Cryer HG, Fildes J. The American College of Surgeons Trauma Quality Improvement Program. Surg Clin 2012;92(2):441.

95. Berian JR, Rosenthal RA, Baker TL, et al. Hospital Standards to Promote Optimal Surgical Care of the Older Adult A Report From the Coalition for Quality in Geriatric Surgery. Ann Surg 2018;267(2):280–90.

Moving?

Make sure your subscription moves with you!

To notify us of your new address, find your **Clinics Account Number** (located on your mailing label above your name), and contact customer service at:

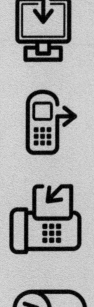

Email: **journalscustomerservice-usa@elsevier.com**

800-654-2452 (subscribers in the U.S. & Canada)
314-447-8871 (subscribers outside of the U.S. & Canada)

Fax number: 314-447-8029

Elsevier Health Sciences Division
Subscription Customer Service
3251 Riverport Lane
Maryland Heights, MO 63043

*To ensure uninterrupted delivery of your subscription, please notify us at least 4 weeks in advance of move.

ELSEVIER

Printed and bound by CPI Group (UK) Ltd, Croydon, CR0 4YY

03/10/2024

01040469-0004